Test Bank

for

Sizer and Whitney's

Nutrition

Concepts and Controversies

Tenth Edition

Jana R. Kicklighter
Georgia State University

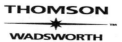

THOMSON

WADSWORTH

Australia • Canada • Mexico • Singapore • Spain • United Kingdom • United States

Printed in the United States of America
2 3 4 5 6 7 08 07 06 05

Printer: Globus

0-534-40676-9

For more information about our products,
contact us at:
Thomson Learning Academic Resource Center
1-800-423-0563

For permission to use material from this text or product, submit a request online at
http://www.thomsonrights.com.
Any additional questions about permissions can be submitted by email to **thomsonrights@thomson.com.**

Thomson Higher Education
10 Davis Drive
Belmont, CA 94002-3098
USA

Asia (including India)
Thomson Learning
5 Shenton Way
#01-01 UIC Building
Singapore 068808

Australia/New Zealand
Thomson Learning Australia
102 Dodds Street
Southbank, Victoria 3006
Australia

Canada
Thomson Nelson
1120 Birchmount Road
Toronto, Ontario M1K 5G4
Canada

UK/Europe/Middle East/Africa
Thomson Learning
High Holborn House
50–51 Bedford Row
London WC1R 4LR
United Kingdom

Latin America
Thomson Learning
Seneca, 53
Colonia Polanco
11560 Mexico
D.F. Mexico

Spain (including Portugal)
Thomson Paraninfo
Calle Magallanes, 25
28015 Madrid, Spain

Table of Contents

Preface iv

Nutrition: Concepts and Controversies **Test Bank** 1
Chapter 1 -   Food Choices and Human Health 1
Chapter 2 -   Nutrition Tools—Standards and Guidelines 9
Chapter 3 -   The Remarkable Body 17
Chapter 4 -   The Carbohydrates: Sugar, Starch, Glycogen, and Fiber..................................24
Chapter 5 -   The Lipids: Fats, Oils, Phospholipids, and Sterols...33
Chapter 6 -   The Proteins and Amino Acids 40
Chapter 7 -   The Vitamins 48
Chapter 8 -   Water and Minerals 56
Chapter 9 -   Energy Balance and Healthy Body Weight..63
Chapter 10 -   Nutrients, Physical Activity, and the Body's Responses....................................70
Chapter 11 -   Diet and Health..78
Chapter 12 -   Food Safety and Food Technology 85
Chapter 13 -   Life Cycle Nutrition: Mother and Infant...93
Chapter 14 -   Child, Teen, and Older Adult 102
Chapter 15 -   Hunger and the Global Environment 110

Telecourse – Nutrition Pathways: Concepts Test Bank..117
    (Contributed by Evelyn Wong)
Lesson 1   Nutrition Basics..117
Lesson 2   The Digestive System 119
Lesson 3   Carbohydrates: Simple and Complex 121
Lesson 4   Carbohydrates: Fiber 122
Lesson 5   Fats: The Lipid Family 124
Lesson 6   Fats: Health Effects 126
Lesson 7   Protein: Form and Function..128
Lesson 8   The Protein Continuum 130
Lesson 9   Metabolism 131
Lesson 10   Weight Control: Energy Regulation..132
Lesson 11   Weight Control: Health Effects 134
Lesson 12   Vitamins: Water-Soluble...137
Lesson 13   Vitamins: Fat-Soluble 138
Lesson 14   Major Minerals and Water...140
Lesson 15   Trace Minerals..143
Lesson 16   Physical Activity: Fitness Basics 146
Lesson 17   Physical Activity: Beyond Fitness...149
Lesson 18   Life Cycle: Pregnancy...151
Lesson 19   Life Cycle: Lactation and Infancy 153
Lesson 20   Life Cycle: Childhood and Adolescence...155

Lesson 21   Life Cycle: Adulthood and Aging...157
Lesson 22   Diet and Health: Cardiovascular Disease 159
Lesson 23   Diet and Health: Cancer, Immunology, and AIDS...161
Lesson 24   Diet and Health: Diabetes 165
Lesson 25   Consumer Concerns and Food Safety 168
Lesson 26   Applied Nutrition 171

Preface

This Test Bank is provided as a supplement to the tenth edition of *Nutrition: Concepts and Controversies*. It includes over 900 test questions. The revised tests for each of the 15 chapters contain a variety of carefully selected items to test the objectives of each chapter and controversy. A variety of item formats are included and questions are designed to test students' comprehension of the material (75%) and their ability to apply important concepts (25%).

Answers and page references, located in the left margin, accompany each multiple-choice, matching, and true/false question. Suggested essay questions, also accompanied by page references, are provided for each chapter. However, essay questions have not been answered since good responses require an analysis and synthesis of knowledge and experiences.

Pages in the Test Bank are perforated and three-hole punched to allow you to arrange your lecture and test material in a sequence that best meets your needs and those of your students. The primary goal of this Test Bank is to assist you in testing important course material and objectives. We hope you will let us hear from you if you find errors or have suggestions for ways to improve the Test Bank.

Jana R. Kicklighter, Ph.D., R.D.
Department of Nutrition
Georgia State University
Atlanta, Georgia 30303

Chapter 1 - Food Choices and Human Health

Ans.	Page	Comprehension Level Items

a   **2**   1.   Malnutrition includes deficiencies, imbalances, and excesses of nutrients, any of which can be detrimental over time.
  a. true
  b. false

c   **3**   2.   Which of the following conditions is the most nutrition responsive?
  a. hypertension
  b. diabetes
  c. iron-deficiency anemia
  d. sickle-cell anemia

b   **7**   3.   The major key to evaluating a food is to:
  a. explore how it can help prevent an illness.
  b. determine how you use it within your total diet over time.
  c. judge how popular it is among consumers.
  d. study the role it plays in the body.

c   **4**   4.   The nutrients fall into _____ classes.
  a. two
  b. four
  c. six
  d. eight

b   **5**   5.   The most energy-rich of the nutrients is:
  a. carbohydrate.
  b. fat.
  c. protein.
  d. water.

a   **4-5**   6.   All of the following nutrients are organic **except:**
  a. minerals.
  b. fat.
  c. vitamins.
  d. carbohydrates.

d   **5**   7.   The energy-yielding nutrients include:
  a. protein.
  b. fat.
  c. vitamins.
  d. a and b
  e. a and c

a   **13**   8.   Once a new finding is published in a scientific journal, it is still only preliminary.
  a. true
  b. false

a   5   9.   Food scientists measure food energy in:
- a.   calories.
- b.   kilograms.
- c.   grams.
- d.   units of weight.

e   5-6   10.   Which of the following are characteristics of alcohol?
- a.   It is a nutrient.
- b.   It contributes calories.
- c.   It interferes with repair of body tissues.
- d.   a and b
- e.   b and c

b   5   11.   Which of the following nutrients yields energy, but also provides materials that form structures and working parts of body tissues?
- a.   carbohydrates
- b.   protein
- c.   fats
- d.   vitamins

c   6   12.   One gram of alcohol is equal to _____ calories.
- a.   two
- b.   four
- c.   seven
- d.   nine

b   5   13.   In nutrition, the word essential means:
- a.   necessary for good health and proper functioning of the body.
- b.   a necessary nutrient that can be obtained only from the diet.
- c.   that the body can manufacture the nutrient from raw materials.
- d.   compounds the body can make for itself.

a   17   14.   Effects of physical activity on the body include all of the following **except:**
- a.   decreased bone density.
- b.   reduced risk of cardiovascular diseases.
- c.   faster wound healing.
- d.   increased lean body tissue.

c   12, 14   15.   The source of valid nutrition information is:
- a.   newspaper articles.
- b.   TV programs.
- c.   scientific journals.
- d.   health magazines.

d   6   16.   The compound that gives hot peppers their burning taste is called a:
- a.   toxin.
- b.   nutrient.
- c.   supplement.
- d.   nonnutrient.

a   6   17.   When a hospital client has to be fed through a vein, the duration should be as short as possible and real food should be reintroduced as early as possible.
- a.   true
- b.   false

d   12   18.   This type of research studies populations and is often used to search for correlations between dietary habits and disease incidence.
- a.   intervention study
- b.   laboratory study
- c.   case study
- d.   epidemiological study

e   12   19.   Which of the following research designs are among the most powerful tools in nutrition research because they show the effects of treatments?
- a.   case study
- b.   laboratory study
- c.   intervention study
- d.   a and b
- e.   b and c

b   17   20.   Heart disease deaths have fallen substantially and the number of overweight people has declined based on evaluation of the nation's progress toward achieving national health objectives.
- a.   true
- b.   false

d   9   21.   A certain amount of fiber in foods contributes to the health of the digestive tract, but too much fiber leads to nutrient losses. The characteristic of diet planning illustrated by this statement is called:
- a.   adequacy.
- b.   calorie control.
- c.   balance.
- d.   moderation.

c   17   22.   Nutrition-related health objectives for the nation have been published by the:
- a.   Department of Agriculture.
- b.   Food and Drug Administration.
- c.   Department of Health and Human Services.
- d.   Centers for Disease Control and Prevention.

b   7   23.   Sugar, butter, and corn oil are examples of _____ foods which provide few nutrients with many calories.
- a.   natural
- b.   partitioned
- c.   processed
- d.   enriched

a   7   24.   Data from a national survey showed that on a given day almost half of our population consume no:
- a.   fruits or fruit juices.
- b.   vegetables.
- c.   grains.
- d.   meat.

a   7   25.   Foods that have been subjected to any process such as addition of additives, milling, or cooking are called_____ foods.
- a.   processed
- b.   partitioned
- c.   natural
- d.   enriched

a 7 26. Enriched and fortified foods are not necessarily more nutritious than whole basic foods.
   a. true
   b. false

c 7 27. Rice is an example of a _____ food used in Southeast Asia.
   a. fortified
   b. natural
   c. staple
   d. processed

a 7 28. Nutraceutical is a term that has no legal definition.
   a. true
   b. false

a 6 29. When used with human beings, elemental diets:
   a. support life.
   b. support optimal growth.
   c. support health.
   d. enable people to thrive.

d 8 30. One of the characteristics of a nutritious diet is that the foods provide enough of each essential nutrient, fiber, and energy. This principle of diet planning is called:
   a. variety.
   b. balance.
   c. moderation.
   d. adequacy.

c 17 31. Successes in meeting the nutrition objectives for the nation as part of *Healthy People 2000* included all of the following **except:**
   a. reductions in incidences of food-borne infections.
   b. reductions in cancers of the breast.
   c. reductions in the number of overweight people.
   d. reductions in infant mortality.

c 3 32. Of the 10 leading causes of death in the United States in 2001, ____ were related to nutrition, and 1 to alcohol consumption.
   a. 2
   b. 3
   c. 4
   d. 5

a 2 33. Malnutrition includes deficiencies, imbalances, and excesses of nutrients.
   a. true
   b. false

d 16 34. According to the *Dietary Guidelines for Americans*, the most healthful diet:
   a. is low in saturated fat.
   b. provides needed fats and oils.
   c. is moderate in cholesterol.
   d. a and b
   e. b and c

b   15   35.   The *Dietary Guidelines for Americans* are intended for adults and healthy children ages
                    _____ and older.
                    a.   one
                    b.   two
                    c.   three
                    d.   four

Application Level Items

a   5   36.   How many calories are in a food that contains 20 grams of carbohydrate, 8 grams
                    protein, and 5 grams of fat?
                    a.   157
                    b.   232
                    c.   258
                    d.   378

a   5   37.   A food provides 8 grams of fat and 300 total calories. What is the percentage of calories
                    as fat in this product?
                    a.   24%
                    b.   30%
                    c.   48%
                    d.   52%

d   19-20 38.   Which of the following foods offers the most nutrients per calorie?
                    a.   potatoes
                    b.   corn
                    c.   green peas
                    d.   carrots

c   6   39.   A compound in cranberries may prevent some bacteria from clinging to the urinary tract
                    and help prevent urinary tract infections. This compound is an example of a:
                    a.   nutraceutical.
                    b.   functional food.
                    c.   phytochemical.
                    d.   natural food.

c   5   40.   Your best friend tells you that she has started taking vitamin supplements to give her
                    energy. How would you respond to her statement?
                    a.   Vitamins are organic and are a great energy source.
                    b.   Vitamins provide energy because they undergo oxidation.
                    c.   Vitamins do not yield usable energy.
                    d.   a and b
                    e.   b and c

d   8-9   41.   Most foods that are high in calcium are poor sources of iron. This statement illustrates
                    the characteristic of a nutritious diet known as:
                    a.   adequacy.
                    b.   variety.
                    c.   moderation.
                    d.   balance.

e   9   42.   Harry has a monotonous diet and eats the same foods every day. You try to convince him to eat a variety of foods because:

    a.   some less well-known nutrients and some nonnutrient food components could be important to health.
    b.   a monotonous diet may deliver large amounts of unwanted toxins or contaminants.
    c.   a monotonous diet may lead to decreased appetite and severe weight loss.
    d.   a and c
    e.   a and b

b   19   43.   Three ounces of beef stew offers about the same amount of iron as three ounces of water-packed tuna, but the beef contains over 300 calories while the tuna contains about 100 calories. This is an example of:

    a.   balance.
    b.   nutrient density.
    c.   dietary variety.
    d.   moderation.

d   13   44.   You see a new finding about nutrition reported in your local newspaper. Based on this information you would:

    a.   decide that the information is factual.
    b.   contribute it to media sensationalism.
    c.   feel confident about changing your diet accordingly.
    d.   wait to apply the findings until they have been repeated and confirmed by scientists.

c   7   45.   You purchase a food product which is enriched. This means that:

    a.   the product is superior to similar products.
    b.   the product is low in calories and high in nutrients.
    c.   the product could be either nutritious or not nutritious.
    d.   a and b
    e.   b and c

b   10   46.   Cultural traditions regarding food are static and inflexible.

    a.   true
    b.   false

a   4   47.   The human genome is 99.9% the same in all people.

    a.   true
    b.   false

b   5   48.   Carbohydrate and protein each contain _____ calories in a gram.

    a.   2
    b.   4
    c.   7
    d.   9

d   7   49.   Which of the following terms was coined in an attempt to identify foods that might lend protection against chronic diseases by way of the nutrients or nonnutrients they contain?

    a.   natural foods
    b.   organic foods
    c.   basic foods
    d.   functional foods

d   15-16   50.   A major guideline for healthy people is to limit calorie intakes and obtain more and varied selections of _____.
  a.   fruits and vegetables
  b.   whole grains
  c.   nonfat or low-fat milk or milk products
  d.   all of the above

Controversy One: Sorting the Imposters from the Real Nutrition Experts

d   23   51.   You can tell a claim about nutrition is suspect if it bears the following characteristics:
  a.   it is being made by an advertiser who is paid to make claims.
  b.   the evidence used to support the claim is in the form of testimonials.
  c.   it appears in a scientific journal which is peer-reviewed.
  d.   a and b
  e.   b and c

a   22   52.   Much of the nutrition information found on the Internet is fiction.
  a.   true
  b.   false

d   24-26   53.   Characteristics of a legitimate and qualified nutrition expert include:
  a.   graduation from a university after completing a program of dietetics.
  b.   completion of an approved internship or the equivalent.
  c.   use of the term nutritionist after the individual's name.
  d.   a and b
  e.   b and c

a   26   54.   The credential R.D. displayed by a dietitian's name indicates registration with:
  a.   the American Dietetic Association.
  b.   the American Association of Nutrition and Dietary Consultants.
  c.   the International Academy of Nutritional Consultants.
  d.   the American Society for Clinical Nutrition.

a   24   55.   Only about a quarter of all medical schools in the United States require students to take even one nutrition course.
  a.   true
  b.   false

a   24, 26   56.   Licensing provides a way to identify people who have met minimum standards of education and experience.
  a.   true
  b.   false

Essay Questions

7   57.   Why does the variety of foods available to us today make it more difficult, rather than easier, to plan nutritious diets?

13   58.   Describe why people should not make changes in their diet based on results of a single research study.

6   59.   Identify the functions of food, in addition to providing nutrients.

8-9   60.   Identify and briefly describe the five characteristics of a nutritious diet.

19-20   61.   Explain the concept of nutrient density and give an example.

22-24   62.   Describe how you would determine if an Internet site offers reliable nutrition information.

17   63.   Describe the potential benefits of physical activity.

10   64.   Identify factors that drive food choices.

11-13   65.   Describe the characteristics of scientific research.

5   66.   Provide some specific examples of how vitamins and minerals serve as regulators in the body.

6   67.   Is it possible to take dietary supplements in place of food? Why or why not?

Ans.	Page	Comprehension Level Items

a   31   1. The Dietary Reference Intakes (DRI) are appropriately used for all of the following **except**:
- a. estimating the nutrient needs of persons with medical problems.
- b. estimating the adequacy of an individual's nutrient intake.
- c. planning diets for population groups like military personnel.
- d. ensuring that minimum nutrient requirements are met.

a   28   2. So far, the DRI Committee has published recommendations for the vitamins and minerals, along with those for carbohydrates, fiber, liquids, proteins and energy.
- a. true
- b. false

b   28   3. Currently, the DRI values for water, the minerals sodium and potassium, and other food constituents are forthcoming.
- a. true
- b. false

d   29   4. Which of the following establishes population-wide average requirements used by nutrition policymakers?
- a. Recommended Dietary Allowances
- b. Daily Values
- c. Recommended Daily Allowances
- d. Estimated Average Requirements

a   33   5. The United States is among many countries which establishes and publishes guidelines for appropriate nutrient intakes.
- a. true
- b. false

b   28, 31   6. Which of the following statements is **not** true about the DRI?
- a. The committee that publishes them is comprised of scientists.
- b. They are minimum requirements, not recommendations.
- c. They are based on review of available scientific research.
- d. They are for individuals who are healthy.

b   30   7. If a nutrient does not have a Tolerable Upper Intake Level, this means that:
- a. it is safe to consume in any amount.
- b. insufficient data exist to establish a value.
- c. no caution is required when consuming supplements of that nutrient.
- d. a and b
- e. b and c

d   33   8. Characteristics of Daily Values include the following:
- a. They apply to all people.
- b. They are ideal for allowing comparisons among foods.
- c. They are useful as nutrient intake goals for individuals.
- d. a and b
- e. a and c

a   31   9.   On average, one should try to get 100% of the DRI for every nutrient to ensure an adequate intake over time.
- a.   true
- b.   false

a   33   10.   The primary difference between recommendations for nutrient intakes and values set for energy intake is that the value for energy intake is not generous.
- a.   true
- b.   false

d   35   11.   Based on the USDA Food Guide, at least ____ of the foods from the fruit group eaten each day should be whole fruits rather than fruit juices.
- a. $^1/_3$
- b.   ¼
- c.   ½
- d. $^2/_3$

d   36   12.   Which of the following foods in the meat, poultry, fish, legumes, eggs, and nuts group of the USDA Food Guide has the highest nutrient density?
- a.   luncheon meats
- b.   fried fish
- c.   duck with skin
- d.   chicken with no skin

a   33   13.   Nutrient contents of packaged foods are stated on food labels as Daily Values.
- a.   true
- b.   false

d   34   14.   Characteristics of food groups plans include all of the following **except:**
- a.   they sort foods into groups based on nutrient content.
- b.   they specify that people should eat certain minimum number of servings from each group.
- c.   the USDA Food Guide utilizes a food group plan.
- d.   they organize foods with respect to their nutrient contents and calorie amounts.

a   33   15.   Many nations and international groups have published sets of standards similar to the DRI.
- a.   true
- b.   false

e   34   16.   The 2005 *Dietary Guidelines* encourage Americans to consume less:
- a.   refined grains.
- b.   fruits.
- c.   added sugars.
- d.   vegetables.
- e.   a and c

b   45   17.   Exchange systems help primarily with:
- a.   balance.
- b.   calorie control.
- c.   adequacy.
- d.   moderation.

c   35-36   18.   Which of the following foods do **not** fit into any of the five major food groups in the USDA Food Guide?
a.   yogurt, legumes, and cheese
b.   peaches, peanuts, and ready-to-eat cereal
c.   margarine, gravy, and jelly
d.   eggs, frozen yogurt, and avocados
e.   macaroni, canned fruit, and vegetable juice

d   34   19.   Food group plans primarily dictate:
a.   particular foods to choose each day.
b.   appropriate portion sizes for foods.
c.   estimates of the amounts of carbohydrate, protein, and fat in foods.
d.   numbers and sizes of servings to choose each day.

b   37-38   20.   All of the following are true regarding the discretionary calorie allowance **except**:
a.   it may be spent on nutrient-dense foods.
b.   the added fat absorbed by the batter in fried chicken does not contribute to discretionary calories.
c.   it may be affected by physical activity level.
d.   it may be spent on added sugars.

c   App. D   21.   In exchange lists, cheese is included as a member of the _____ list.
a.   milk
b.   vegetable
c.   meat
d.   fat

b   41   22.   One of the major disadvantages of the USDA Food Guide is that it cannot be adapted to other national and cultural cuisines.
a.   true
b.   false

d   37   23.   The best way for a person to get all the essential nutrients and keep energy intake low is to:
a.   use the principle of the discretionary calorie allowance to plan their diet.
b.   choose foods with high nutrient density in each food group.
c.   follow the principle of moderation in dietary intake.
d.   a and b
e.   a and c

c   45   24.   All of the following are characteristics of exchange systems **except**:
a.   they pay special attention to calories.
b.   they give a sense of which foods are similar to each other.
c.   they sort foods by their carbohydrate contents only.
d.   they highlight the fact that most foods provide more than just one energy nutrient.

b   App. D   25.   In the exchange lists, milk is categorized according to:
a.   the type of fat.
b.   fat content.
c.   protein content.
d.   calcium content.

App. D 26. Match the exchange lists on the right with the amount of energy nutrients they contain listed on the left.

	CHO	PRO	FAT		
e	___ 15	3	0-1	a.	lean meat
g	___ -	7	8	b.	vegetable
c	___ 12	8	0-3	c.	nonfat milk
d	___ -	-	5	d.	fat
b	___ 5	2	-	e.	starch
a	___ -	7	3	f.	fruit
f	___ 15	-	-	g.	high-fat meat
i	___ -	7	5	h.	whole milk
h	___ 12	8	8	i.	medium-fat meat
j	___ 12	8	5	j.	low-fat milk

a 45 27. The exchange list system highlights the fact that many meats contain more calories from fat than from protein.
   a. true
   b. false

d 47 28. Which of the following foods is exempt from listing ingredients on the label?
   a. mayonnaise
   b. salad dressing
   c. ice cream
   d. none of the above

d 36 29. In the USDA Food Guide, one ounce of meat is equal to all of the following **except:**
   a. 1 oz. cooked fish.
   b. 1 egg.
   c. 1 tbs. peanut butter.
   d. ½ cup cooked legumes.

e 49 30. Amounts of these types of lipids must be listed on food labels:
   a. monounsaturated fat.
   b. *trans* fat.
   c. cholesterol.
   d. a and b
   e. b and c

c 49-50 31. Any food providing 10% or more of the Daily Value for a nutrient is considered to be a _____ source of the nutrient.
   a. poor
   b. reliable
   c. good
   d. excellent

e 31 32. The DRI are defined for:
   a. health maintenance.
   b. restoration of health.
   c. disease prevention.
   d. a and b
   e. a and c

b	33	33.	The Daily Values reflect the needs of an "average person" consuming between _____ and _____ calories a day.

    a.   1,500 and 2,000
    b.   2,000 and 2,500
    c.   2,500 and 3,000
    d.   3,000 and 3,500

d   47   34.   The bottom portion of the Nutrition Facts panel on a food package:
    a.   is identical on every label.
    b.   lists the Daily Values standards.
    c.   conveys information specific to the food inside the package.
    d.   a and b
    e.   b and c

a   49   35.   The percentages of the Daily Values on food packages are given in terms of a person requiring _____ calories each day.
    a.   2,000
    b.   2,500
    c.   3,000
    d.   3,500

b   30   36.   The absence of a Tolerable Upper Intake Level for a nutrient implies that it is safe to consume in any amount.
    a.   true
    b.   false

c   30   37.   The DRI Committee recommended a diet that contains _____% of its calories from carbohydrate.
    a.   10-35
    b.   20-35
    c.   45-65
    d.   50-70

c   34-37   38.   Which of the following groups is de-emphasized in the USDA Food Guide?
    a.   vegetables
    b.   fruits
    c.   meats
    d.   grains

a   37   39.   Which vegetable subgroup of the USDA Food Guide is not correctly matched with its target nutrient(s)?
    a.   orange and deep yellow vegetables – vitamin D
    b.   starchy vegetables – carbohydrate
    c.   dark green vegetables – folate
    d.   legumes – iron and protein

Application Level Items

c   30-31   40.   Which of the following people would **not** be covered by the DRI, based on assumptions made by the DRI committee?
    a.   Harry, a 35 year old healthy businessman
    b.   Cindy, a 21 year old college athlete
    c.   Robert, a 20 year old with cystic fibrosis
    d.   Joann, a 35 year old female vegetarian

b   48   41.   If a food label states that a food contains eight percent of the Daily Value for dietary fiber, the food would contain _____ grams of dietary fiber per serving.
a.   one
b.   two
c.   three
d.   four

c   30   42.   George is a 35-year-old athlete using nutrient supplements to give him a competitive advantage. Which of the following nutrient intake recommendations would you suggest that George become familiar with?
a.   Adequate Intakes
b.   Estimated Average Requirements
c.   Tolerable Upper Intake Levels
d.   Recommended Dietary Allowances

e   47-51   43.   You are speaking to a group of consumers about ways to use food labels to choose healthy foods in the grocery store. During your presentation, you would emphasize the following:
a.   using the grams and numbers on the labels to calculate percentages.
b.   comparing similar food products on nutrient components.
c.   understanding the descriptive terms used on food labels.
d.   a and b
e.   b and c

b   35,36,39   44.   Which of the following includes the recommended daily amounts of food from each group for a sedentary woman of 32 who requires 1,800 kcal/day, based on the USDA Food Guide?
a.   1 cup nonfat milk; 1 slice toast; ½ cup oatmeal; ¾ cup orange juice; 3 oz. chicken breast; ½ cup green beans; 1 medium apple
b.   ½ cup grape juice; 2 tbs. peanut butter on 2 slices whole wheat bread; 1 cup nonfat yogurt; 1 medium apple; ½ cup diced cucumbers; 3 oz. baked fish; 1 cup spinach leaves; 1 cup squash; ½ cup carrots; 1 cup cooked rice; 2-oz. whole wheat dinner roll; ½ cup strawberries; 2 cups nonfat milk
c.   1 cup nonfat milk; 1 cup raisin bran; 1 medium apricot; 1 egg; 3 oz. steak; 1 medium baked potato; ½ cup broccoli; 1 cup nonfat milk; 2-oz. whole wheat roll
d.   2 slices whole wheat bread with 1 ½ oz. fat-free natural cheese; ½ cup apple juice; 3 oz. tuna fish salad with 1 cup lettuce leaves; 1 oz. crackers; 1 cup milk; 3 oz. pork chop; ½ cup Brussels sprouts; ½ cup fruit cocktail

c   App. D   45.   How many calories are in a meal pattern that provides 1 starch exchange, 1 fruit exchange, 1 nonfat milk exchange, and 1 lean meat exchange for breakfast?
a.   200
b.   250
c.   285
d.   300

b   45   46.   If you were teaching someone with diabetes how to plan a diet to control carbohydrate intakes, which of the following tools would you use?
a.   the USDA Food Guide
b.   the exchange list system
c.   the Healthy Eating Index
d.   *Dietary Guidelines for Americans*

d   47   47.   If vitamin C has been added to cranberry juice, the label must include:

    a.   nutrient information.

    b.   an ingredients list.

    c.   a health claim.

    d.   a and b

    e.   b and c

c   48   48.   The Nutrition Facts Panel on a food label lists the following information for amounts per serving: 111 calories; 23 calories from fat. What percentage of the calories are provided by fat?

    a.   11%

    b.   19%

    c.   21%

    d.   32%

Controversy Two – Phytochemicals and Functional Foods: What Do they Promise? What Do they Deliver?

a   57   49.   Which of the following is the best and safest source of phytochemicals?

    a.   whole foods

    b.   supplements

    c.   herbal remedies

    d.   organic foods

d   59   50.   Which phytochemical is contained in whole grains, fruits, vegetables, herbs, spices, teas and red wine?

    a.   carotenoids

    b.   lignans

    c.   lutein

    d.   flavonoids

c   60   51.   Compared to people in the West, Asians suffer less frequently from all of the following **except:**

    a.   osteoporosis.

    b.   heart disease.

    c.   stomach cancer.

    d.   symptoms related to menopause.

a   61   52.   One of the best sources of lycopene is:

    a.   tomatoes.

    b.   soy products.

    c.   garlic.

    d.   flaxseed.

Essay Questions

31-32   53.   Describe how the DRI Committee establishes DRI values.

33   54.   Differentiate between the methods used in setting the recommended intake for nutrients versus the recommended energy intake values.

33, 49   55.   Describe characteristics of the Daily Values listed on food labels and how they should be used in diet planning.

45   56.   Identify the specific advantages of exchange systems.

34-37   57.   List the major groups and subgroups of the USDA Food Guide, and give an example of a nutrient-dense food from each.

37-38   58.   Explain the concept of the discretionary calorie allowance, and describe ways this allowance may be "spent."

34   59.   Identify the American College of Sports Medicine's recommendations for daily physical activity.

61-62   60.   Defend the statement in the controversy that foods, not supplements, are the best and safest source of phytochemicals.

Chapter 3 – The Remarkable Body

Ans.	Page	**Comprehension Level Items**

c   66   1.   Cells can best be described as:
- a.   the basis of the body's design.
- b.   the vital components of foods.
- c.   self-contained living entities.
- d.   building blocks of the body.

a   68   2.   Cells are organized into tissues that perform specialized tasks and tissues, in turn, are grouped together to form whole organs.
- a.   true
- b.   false

d   66   3.   Among the cells' most basic needs are _____ and the oxygen with which to burn it.
- a.   water
- b.   essential nutrients
- c.   building blocks
- d.   energy

a   66   4.   The first principle of diet planning is that the foods we choose must provide energy and the essential nutrients, including:
- a.   water.
- b.   fuel.
- c.   oxygen.
- d.   carbon dioxide.

d   67   5.   Which of the following determines the nature of the cell's work?
- a.   organs
- b.   mutations
- c.   red blood cells
- d.   genes

a   68   6.   Body fluids supply the tissues continuously with energy, oxygen and nutrients, including water.
- a.   true
- b.   false

e   68   7.   The body's main fluid(s) is (are):
- a.   intracellular fluid.
- b.   blood.
- c.   lymph.
- d.   a and b
- e.   b and c

d   68   8.   The blood picks up oxygen and releases carbon dioxide in the:
- a.   heart.
- b.   liver.
- c.   digestive system.
- d.   lungs.

a	66-67	9.	Cells lining the digestive tract replace themselves every:			
			a.	3 days.		
			b.	2 weeks.		
			c.	4 months.		
			d.	12 months.		

b   71   10.   When the pancreas detects a high concentration of the blood's sugar, glucose, it releases:
a.   lymph.
b.   insulin.
c.   antibodies.
d.   glucagon.

c   71   11.   Hormones are secreted and released into the blood by _____.
a.   antigens
b.   enzymes
c.   glands
d.   antibodies

a   73   12.   Which of the following are the first to defend the body tissues against invaders?
a.   phagocytes
b.   antigens
c.   T-cells
d.   B-cells

c   73   13.   Which of the following does **not** occur as part of the stress response?
a.   The muscles tense up.
b.   The liver pours forth glucose from its stores.
c.   The digestive system speeds up.
d.   The fat cells release fat.

d   72   14.   Which of the following alert(s) your conscious mind to the sensation of hunger?
a.   brain
b.   hormones
c.   taste buds
d.   a and b
e.   b and c

15.   Match the digestive organs, listed on the left, with their appropriate functions, listed on the right.

i	76	_____ mouth	a.	manufactures bile to help digest fats
g	76	_____ esophagus	b.	conducts bile into the small intestine
d	76	_____ stomach	c.	opens to allow elimination
k	76	_____ small intestine	d.	churns, mixes, and grinds food to a liquid mass
a	76	_____ liver	e.	reabsorbs water and minerals
f	76	_____ gallbladder	f.	stores bile until needed
h	76	_____ pancreas	g.	passes food to stomach
e	76	_____ large intestine	h.	manufacturers enzymes to digest all energy-yielding nutrients
j	76	_____ rectum	i.	chews and mixes foods with saliva
c	76	_____ anus	j	stores waste prior to elimination
			k.	secretes enzymes that digest carbohydrate, fat, and protein

b 78 16. The digestive tract needs _____ that provides the bulk against which the muscles of the colon can work.
    a. energy
    b. fiber
    c. nutrients
    d. water

e 88 17. The liver converts excess energy-containing nutrients into:
    a. glycogen.
    b. protein.
    c. fat.
    d. a and b
    e. a and c

b 72 18. The nervous system's role in hunger regulation is coordinated by the:
    a. pancreas.
    b. brain.
    c. digestive tract.
    d. spinal cord.

c 79 19. The primary organ of digestion and absorption is the:
    a. mouth.
    b. stomach.
    c. small intestine.
    d. large intestine.

a 68-69 20. Which of the following has the special task of chemically altering absorbed materials to make them better suited for use by other tissues?
    a. liver
    b. pancreas
    c. stomach
    d. small intestine

d 88 21. Which of the following is(are) characteristic(s) of liver glycogen?
    a. It is stored for the body's ongoing glucose needs.
    b. It can be released into the blood as glucose.
    c. It can store up to a three-day supply of glycogen.
    d. a and b
    e. b and c

b 88 22. Without food to replenish it, the liver's glycogen supply can be depleted within:
    a. 1 - 3 hours.
    b. 3 - 6 hours.
    c. 4 - 8 hours.
    d. 6 - 9 hours.

b 88 23. The bones provide reserves of:
    a. vitamins.
    b. calcium.
    c. glycogen.
    d. a and b
    e. b and c

a	88	24.	Some nutrients are stored in the body in much smaller quantities than others are. a. true b. false

d	88	25.	Which of the following is **not** one of the major storage systems which store and release nutrients to meet the cells' needs between meals? a. liver b. muscles c. fat cells d. pancreas

c	66-67	26.	Which of the following cells replace themselves every three days? a. muscle b. skin c. digestive tract d. red blood

d	74	27.	Most people have aversions to _____ tastes. a. sweet b. salty c. fatty d. bitter

b	77	28.	Chewing food for an extended time provides additional advantages to digestion. a. true b. false

a	79	29.	The stomach's main function is the digestion of this nutrient: a. protein. b. carbohydrate. c. fat. d. fiber.

b	79	30.	Timing of meals is important because the digestive tract is unable to digest food at certain times. a. true b. false

d	67	31.	Which of the following types of cells do not reproduce, and if damaged by injury or disease, are lost forever? a. skin cells b. red blood cells c. muscle cells d. brain cells

b	74	32.	Which of the following poses a formidable obstacle to a successful organ transplant? a. phagocytes b. T-cells c. B-cells d. antibodies

a	88	33.	Some vitamins are stored in the body without limit, even if they reach toxic levels. a. true b. false

Application Level Items

d   86-87   34.   Which of the following advice would you give to a friend suffering from constipation?
- a.   Consume foods with adequate fiber.
- b.   Drink enough water.
- c.   Take a laxative.
- d.   a and b
- e.   b and c

b   72-73   35.   A person can eat when hunger is absent because:
- a.   the hypothalamus monitors the availability of nutrients.
- b.   the conscious mind of the cortex can override body signals.
- c.   the digestive tract sends messages to the hypothalamus.
- d.   the stomach intensifies its contractions and creates hunger pangs.

a   71, 79   36.   You have just consumed a meal very high in fat. As a result, hormonal messages will tell an organ to send _____ in amounts matched to the amount of fat present.
- a.   bile
- b.   bicarbonate
- c.   hydrochloric acid
- d.   mucus

c   83   37.   Which of the following would occur in a malnourished child?
- a.   The absorptive surface of the small intestine would increase in size.
- b.   The absorptive surface of the small intestine would become more efficient at its job.
- c.   The absorptive surface of the small intestine would shrink.
- d.   a and b
- e.   b and c

a   88   38.   A person in an emergency situation is unable to eat for several weeks. Which of the following would provide the energy which this person would need to survive?
- a.   fat
- b.   liver glycogen
- c.   bones
- d.   muscle glycogen

d   79   39.   Which of the following statements is true regarding the timing of meals?
- a.   Timing of meals is important because the digestive tract is unable to digest foods at certain times.
- b.   A meal should be consumed immediately before exercise to enhance physical work.
- c.   Eating a meal late at night is desirable because it facilitates sleep.
- d.   Timing of meals is important to feeling well.

d   85   40.   Which of the following strategies should be used by someone experiencing heartburn?
- a.   Drink liquids an hour before or after meals.
- b.   Eat smaller meals.
- c.   Lie down after meals.
- d.   a and b
- e.   b and c

d   88   41.   Which of the following should be consumed at intervals throughout the day?
- a.   vitamin-rich foods
- b.   fat-containing foods
- c.   mineral-rich foods
- d.   carbohydrate-containing foods

Controversy Three: Alcohol and Nutrition: Do the Benefits Outweigh the Risks?

e   93   42.   Which of the following deliver one-half ounce of ethanol?
- a.   5 ounces of wine
- b.   2 ounces hard liquor
- c.   12 ounces beer
- d.   a and b
- e.   a and c

a   93   43.   A person can become intoxicated almost immediately when drinking, especially if:
- a.   the stomach is empty.
- b.   drinks are consumed quickly.
- c.   carbohydrate snacks are consumed at the same time.
- d.   the drink is not diluted with water.

c   94   44.   Which of the following organs makes almost all of the body's alcohol-processing machinery?
- a.   stomach
- b.   pancreas
- c.   liver
- d.   spleen

a   95   45.   Which of the following restores sobriety in someone who has been drinking alcohol?
- a.   time
- b.   walking
- c.   drinking coffee
- d.   eating food

b   95   46.   Alcohol affects body functions in all of the following ways **except:**
- a.   alters amino acid metabolism.
- b.   slows down the synthesis of fatty acids.
- c.   weakens the body's defenses against infection.
- d.   causes symptoms like those of gout.

Essay Questions

71-72   47.   Describe how hormones affect nutrition.

69-70   48.   Identify and describe three factors necessary to ensure efficient circulation of fluid to all body cells.

73   49.   Describe what happens during the stress response and the possible consequences for people living in the modern world.

81-82   50.   How would you respond to a friend's statement that people should not consume fruit and meat at the same meal?

73-74   51.   Briefly describe the actions of the body's phagocytes and lymphocytes.

77-80   52.   Differentiate between the mechanical and chemical aspects of digestion.

83   53.   Describe what happens to digestion and absorption in cases of severe undernutrition.

88   54.   Explain why sources of carbohydrate should be consumed at intervals throughout the day.

97   55.   Explain why nutrient deficiencies are an inevitable consequence of alcohol abuse.

97, 98   56.   What advice would you give to someone interested in improving her appetite with alcohol?

Chapter 4 - The Carbohydrates
Sugar, Starch, Glycogen, and Fiber

Ans.	Page	Comprehension Level Items

Comprehension Level Items

c   100

1. Which of the following animal-derived foods contains significant amounts of carbohydrates?
   - a. eggs
   - b. beef
   - c. milk
   - d. poultry

c   102

2. Complex carbohydrates:
   - a. include both single sugar units and linked pairs of sugar units.
   - b. are known as the monosaccharides and disaccharides.
   - c. are long chains of sugar units arranged to form starch or fiber.
   - d. a and b
   - e. b and c

b   100

3. Which of the following monosaccharides is responsible for the sweet taste of fruit?
   - a. glucose
   - b. fructose
   - c. galactose
   - d. sucrose

a   101

4. When fructose and glucose are bonded together they form:
   - a. table sugar.
   - b. malt sugar.
   - c. milk sugar.
   - d. fruit sugar.

c   101

5. Which of the following is the most-used monosaccharide inside the body?
   - a. fructose
   - b. lactose
   - c. glucose
   - d. galactose

d   101

6. The disaccharides include:
   - a. sucrose, galactose, and maltose.
   - b. maltose, fructose, and galactose.
   - c. lactose, glucose, and fructose.
   - d. sucrose, maltose, and lactose.

7. Match the disaccharides listed on the right with their monosaccharide constituents, listed on the left.

b   101   _____ fructose + glucose   a. maltose

c   101   _____ glucose + galactose   b. sucrose

a   101   _____ glucose + glucose   c. lactose

d 101,125-126 8. Fruits differ from concentrated sweets because:
      a.   their sugars are diluted in large volumes of water.
      b.   they are packaged with fiber.
      c.   they are less nutrient dense.
      d.   a and b
      e.   b and c

c 100-102 9. Which of the following is **not** one of the complex carbohydrates?
      a.   most fibers
      b.   glycogen
      c.   galactose
      d.   starch

a 102 10. The best known fibers include all of the following **except:**
      a.   glycogen.
      b.   cellulose.
      c.   hemicellulose.
      d.   pectin.

c 103 11. Which of the following is **not** an example of fiber?
      a.   "strings" of celery
      b.   membranes surrounding kernels of wheat
      c.   residue in milk
      d.   skins of corn kernels

d 102 footnote 12. The Committee on DRI recently came up with the term total fiber, which includes:
      a.   dietary fiber.
      b.   functional fiber.
      c.   crude fiber.
      d.   a and b
      e.   b and c

c 104 13. Which of the following is the preferred fuel for most body functions?
      a.   protein
      b.   ketones
      c.   carbohydrate
      d.   fat

b 104-105 14. Carbohydrate has been rightly accused of being the fattening ingredient of foods; therefore, we need to consume fewer starchy foods.
      a.   true
      b.   false

d 105 15. Current dietary guidelines for the United States recommend:
      a.   restricted intake of carbohydrates for diabetic clients.
      b.   increased consumption of all kinds of carbohydrates.
      c.   reduction in both simple and complex carbohydrate intakes.
      d.   increased consumption of fiber-rich, whole food sources of carbohydrate.

a 106-109 16. Which of the following is **not** an effect of fiber?
      a.   promotes weight gain and feeling of fullness
      b.   prevents constipation and hemorrhoids
      c.   reduces the risks of heart and artery disease
      d.   prevents appendicitis and diverticulosis

a   109   17. Most unrefined plant foods contain a mix of fiber types.
     a.   true
     b.   false

c   106   18. Which of the following foods would you choose as an effective stool-softening agent?
     a.   oat bran
     b.   carrots
     c.   wheat bran
     d.   legumes

d   106-107   19. Which of the following foods has the greatest cholesterol lowering effect?
     a.   wheat bran
     b.   apples
     c.   legumes
     d.   oat bran

d   112-113   20. Potential harmful effects of too much fiber include:
     a.   dehydration.
     b.   limits the absorption of iron.
     c.   extreme weight loss.
     d.   a and b
     e.   b and c

b   109   21. A desirable intake of dietary fiber is _____ grams daily, according to the American Dietetic Association.
     a.   10 - 26
     b.   20 - 35
     c.   27 - 40
     d.   40 - 55

d   109, 113   22. The best way to achieve a desirable amount of fiber is to:
     a.   include fruits, vegetables, and grains in the diet.
     b.   emphasize whole, unprocessed foods.
     c.   add purified fibers to foods.
     d.   a and b
     e.   a and c

d   106   23. Which of the following is **not** a major source of soluble fiber?
     a.   fruits
     b.   legumes
     c.   vegetables
     d.   brown rice

a   106   24. All of the following are health benefits of insoluble fiber **except**:
     a.   lowers risk of diabetes.
     b.   alleviates constipation.
     c.   lowers risk of hemorrhoids.
     d.   may help with weight management.

c   110-111   25. Which of the following nutrients is **not** required by law to be added to refined grain products?
- a. riboflavin
- b. folate
- c. magnesium
- d. thiamin
- e. niacin

b   111   26. The term *"brown bread"* on a label is a guarantee that the bread has been made with whole-grain flour.
- a. true
- b. false

a   113   27. Digestion of most starch begins in the:
- a. mouth.
- b. esophagus.
- c. stomach.
- d. small intestine.

d   117   28. Which of the following statements is **false** concerning the splitting of glucose for energy?
- a. Inside a cell glucose is broken in half and these two halves have two pathways open to them.
- b. Glucose can be broken down to yield energy and carbon dioxide.
- c. Glucose fragments can be hitched together into units of body fat.
- d. Body fat can be converted into glucose to feed the brain adequately.

c   117   29. Products of the incomplete breakdown of fat when carbohydrates are not available are called:
- a. protein-sparing products.
- b. glycogen bodies.
- c. ketone bodies.
- d. glucagon products.

d   117-118   30. Approximately _____ grams a day of carbohydrate are needed to ensure complete sparing of body protein in an average-size person.
- a. 50
- b. 75
- c. 100
- d. 130

a   118   31. When the blood glucose level rises after a meal, the first organ to respond is the:
- a. pancreas.
- b. liver.
- c. stomach.
- d. gallbladder.

b   119   32. The extent to which a food raises the blood glucose level and elicits an insulin response as compared with pure glucose can be measured and ranked on a scale called the:
- a. digestibility index.
- b. glycemic index.
- c. hypoglycemic index.
- d. insulin index.

a   119   33. The glycemic index and glycemic load of foods may be important to people with diabetes who must strive to regulate blood glucose control.
         a.   true
         b.   false

d   121   34. Characteristics of type 1 diabetes include:
         a.   the person's immune system attacks the cells of the pancreas.
         b.   the pancreas no longer produces insulin.
         c.   the person is usually overweight.
         d.   a and b
         e.   b and c

a   123   35. Which of the following helps prevent type 2 diabetes?
         a.   weight control, exercise, and a healthy lifestyle
         b.   taking oral hypoglycemic agents
         c.   restricting protein intake
         d.   watching caffeine intake

c   125   36. With two exceptions, the following food group provides almost no carbohydrate to the diet:
         a.   milk, cheese and yogurt.
         b.   grains.
         c.   meat, poultry, fish, dry beans, eggs and nuts.
         d.   vegetables.

b   105   37. According to the Dietary Reference Intakes, people should obtain about _____ percent of their daily energy from carbohydrates.
         a.   40 - 55
         b.   45 - 65
         c.   50 - 65
         d.   50 - 75

c   122   38. Characteristics of type 2 diabetes include all of the following **except:**
         a.   insulin resistance of the body's cells.
         b.   blood glucose levels rise too high.
         c.   pancreas makes too little or no insulin.
         d.   blood insulin levels rise too high.

c   113   39. All of the following groups are particularly vulnerable to harmful effects of consuming too much fiber **except:**
         a.   the elderly.
         b.   the malnourished.
         c.   adults.
         d.   children who consume no animal products.

b   111   40. Which of the following terms would you look for on a bread label to choose the most nutritious product?
         a.   wheat flour
         b.   whole grain
         c.   unbleached flour
         d.   brown bread

a   116   41. Which of the following would be the best calcium source for an adult with milk allergy?
            a.   canned salmon with bones
            b.   aged cheese
            c.   orange juice
            d.   yogurt

d   122   42. A friend complains of blurred vision, cravings for sweets, weakness, and excessive thirst
            and urination. These symptoms are suggestive of:
            a.   lactose intolerance.
            b.   fasting.
            c.   hypoglycemia.
            d.   diabetes.

e   123   43. The best diet for managing diabetes:
            a.   provides the recommended amount of fiber.
            b.   is low in concentrated sugar.
            c.   is adequate in protein.
            d.   a and b
            e.   a and c

d   125   44. About 15 grams of carbohydrate are found in which of the following?
            a.   a slice of bread
            b.   ½ cup of cooked corn
            c.   1 cup of dried fruit
            d.   a and b
            e.   b and c

e   129   45. To magnify the sweetness of foods without boosting their calories, you would:
            a.   serve sweet food warm.
            b.   reduce the sugar added to recipes by one-half.
            c.   use small amounts of sugar substitutes in place of sucrose.
            d.   a and b
            e.   a and c

b   104   46. The best way to lose fat, maintain lean body tissues, and maintain the health of the body
            is to:
            a.   control calories from fat.
            b.   control total calories.
            c.   control calories from carbohydrate.
            d.   control calories from protein.

Application Level Items

b   101   47. One of your friends makes the statement that her diet contains no sucrose because she
            does not consume table sugar. What would be an appropriate response to this statement?
            a.   You're right, because sucrose is only found in table sugar.
            b.   You're wrong, because sucrose occurs naturally in many fruits and vegetables.
            c.   You're wrong, because sucrose occurs in germinating seeds and arises during
                    digestion.
            d.   You're wrong, because sucrose is found in milk.

d   102   48. Plants store sucrose as starch because:
- a.   glucose is soluble in water.
- b.   the glucose would be washed away by rain.
- c.   glucose is insoluble in water.
- d.   a and b
- e.   b and c

d   104-105   49. You are trying to convince someone that a low-carbohydrate diet is undesirable. Reasons you would give to support your statement include:
- a.   fat is not normally used as fuel by the brain and nervous system.
- b.   gram for gram, carbohydrates donate fewer calories than dietary fats.
- c.   low-carbohydrate diets are expensive and require the purchase of special foods.
- d.   a and b
- e.   a and c

e   109   50. It would be appropriate to recommend high-fiber foods to someone trying to lose weight because:
- a.   it speeds up movement of foods through the upper digestive tract.
- b.   it promotes a feeling of fullness.
- c.   it may displace calorie-dense concentrated fats.
- d.   a and b
- e.   b and c

b   106   51. You are teaching a client how to possibly lower blood cholesterol levels by consuming foods high in fiber. Which of the following foods would be **least** effective for this purpose?
- a.   oat bran cereals
- b.   whole wheat breads
- c.   carrots
- d.   legumes

e   111   52. How would you respond to someone who states that white bread is just as nutritious as whole wheat bread?
- a.   White bread is just as nutritious because it has been enriched with iron, niacin, riboflavin, thiamin, and folate.
- b.   Whole wheat bread is preferable because it is likely to contain several nutrients not added to white bread.
- c.   Whole wheat bread is higher in fiber content than white bread.
- d.   a and b
- e.   b and c

c   113   53. After chewing a piece of bread for awhile, you begin to experience a slightly sweet taste. This taste results from:
- a.   sucrose used in making bread.
- b.   an abnormal use of the carbohydrate in bread.
- c.   the liberation of maltose from starch.
- d.   one of the symptoms of diabetes.

e   116   54. Which of the following would you recommend for a person with lactose intolerance?
- a.   milk
- b.   aged cheese
- c.   yogurt
- d.   a and b
- e.   b and c

d	124	55. Which of the following would be appropriate to try if you experience symptoms of postprandial hypoglycemia? a. Eat regularly timed meals. b. Consume balanced meals that contain protein. c. Deprive your system of carbohydrates. d. a and b e. a and c
d	120	56. What recommendations would you provide to someone trying to improve his workout? a. Eat a small snack rich in complex carbohydrates two hours before the workout. b. Drink some extra fluid before the workout. c. Avoid caffeine-containing beverages before the workout. d. a and b e. b and c

Controversy Four: Sugar and Alternative Sweeteners: Are They Bad for You?

b	132	57. Which of the following is most closely related to diabetes? a. sugar content of the diet b. body fatness c. fat content of the diet d. lean body tissue
a	134	58. Populations with diets with no more than 10 percent of calories from sugar have a low prevalence of dental caries. a. true b. false
c	134	59. Whether or not a food is likely to result in dental caries depends on all of the following **except:** a. how sticky the food is. b. how often it is consumed. c. the bacterial content of the food. d. the length of time the food stays in the mouth.
b	137	60. Which of the following artificial sweeteners is made from sucrose? a. aspartame b. sucralose c. saccharin d. acesulfame-K
a	138	61. Current evidence indicates that moderate intakes of artificial sweeteners pose no health risks. a. true b. false
c	136-137	62. Which of the following synthetic sweeteners should **not** be given to individuals with phenylketonuria? a. saccharin b. sucralose c. aspartame d. neotame

112-113   63. Describe the harmful effects of fiber when taken in excess.

113-115   64. Describe the tasks of the various body systems in breaking down carbohydrate into glucose to fuel the cells' work.

117   65. Explain what is meant by the protein-sparing action of carbohydrate.

124   66. Differentiate between the definitions and symptoms of postprandial hypoglycemia and fasting hypoglycemia.

122   67. Explain the relationship between obesity and type 2 diabetes.

114   68. What advice would you give to someone who desires to increase fiber intake without experiencing problems with gas?

104-105   69. Explain why, calorie for calorie, carbohydrate-rich foods contribute less to body fatness than do fat-rich foods.

134   70. Why don't sugar alcohols contribute to dental caries?

131   71. What accounts for the steady upward trend in U.S. sugar consumption?

Chapter 5 - The Lipids
Fats, Oils, Phospholipids, and Sterols

Ans.	Page	Comprehension Level Items

Comprehension Level Items

b   140

1. A family of organic compounds soluble in organic solvents but not in water is called:
   a. triglycerides.
   b. lipids.
   c. fats.
   d. oils.

2. Match the fat-related terms on the right to their appropriate definitions on the left.

d   140   _____ a lipid that is solid at room temperature   a. cholesterol

e   140   _____ one of the three main classes of dietary lipids; chief form of fat in foods   b. phospholipid

        c. sterol

f   140   _____ a phospholipid which is a major constituent of cell membranes   d. fat

        e. triglyceride

a   140   _____ one of the sterols manufactured in the body   f. lecithin

c   140   _____ one of the three main classes of lipids with a structure similar to cholesterol   g. oil

b   140   _____ one of the three main classes of lipids which is similar to a triglyceride

g   140   _____ a lipid that is liquid at room temperature

a   140

3. About 95% of the lipids in foods and in the human body are:
   a. triglycerides.
   b. phospholipids.
   c. sterols.
   d. cholesterol.

c   140

4. Cholesterol is the best known of the:
   a. phospholipids.
   b. lipids.
   c. sterols.
   d. triglycerides.

c   151

5. The main dietary factor associated with elevated blood cholesterol is:
   a. high cholesterol intake.
   b. high food fat intake.
   c. high saturated and *trans* fat intake.
   d. high polyunsaturated fat intake.

d   161

6. Foods with hidden fat include:
   a. coconuts.
   b. biscuits.
   c. fat on a steak.
   d. a and b
   e. b and c

b   141   7. All of the following are found mainly in foods that contain fat **except:**
- a. vitamin A.
- b. vitamin B_{12}.
- c. vitamin D.
- d. vitamin K.

c   141   8. Which of the following is **not** a function of fat in the human body?
- a. protects the body from temperature extremes
- b. cushions the internal organs from physical shock
- c. carries the water-soluble nutrients
- d. provides the major material from which cell membranes are made

d   142   9. Fatty acids may differ from one another:
- a. in chain length.
- b. in degree of saturation.
- c. in number of calories.
- d. a and b
- e. b and c

e   158   10. Vegetable oils comprise most of the added fat in the diet because:
- a. fast food chains use them for frying.
- b. consumers prefer their taste.
- c. food manufacturers add them to processed foods.
- d. a and b
- e. a and c

e   154   11. Characteristics of the essential fatty acids include:
- a. they must be supplied by the diet.
- b. they can be made from the substances in the body.
- c. they are polyunsaturated fatty acids.
- d. b and c
- e. a and c

b   155-156   12. Consuming _____ fish meals a week will result in the right balance between omega-3 and omega-6 intakes.
- a. 1-2
- b. 2-3
- c. 3-4
- d. 4-5

d   158   13. Cooking oils should be stored in tightly covered containers in order to:
- a. prevent them from becoming rancid.
- b. retard the oxidation process.
- c. prevent them from losing fat soluble vitamins.
- d. a and b
- e. a and c

c   159   14. BHA and BHT are examples of:
- a. hydrogenated fats.
- b. unsaturated fatty acids.
- c. antioxidants.
- d. snack foods.

a   142   15. Fatty acids in foods influence the composition of fats in the body.
- a. true
- b. false

c   155   16. EPA and DHA are:
- a. not important in nutrition.
- b. essential fatty acids.
- c. found in the oils of fish.
- d. omega-6 fatty acids.

d   158   17. Which of the following is(are) characteristic(s) of spreadable margarines made from polyunsaturated oils?
- a. Hydrogen is forced into the oil and some of the unsaturated fatty acids accept it.
- b. The oil becomes harder after the hydrogen is added.
- c. The margarine becomes less saturated than the original oil.
- d. a and b
- e. b and c

a   158-160   18. The most heart healthy margarines are those:
- a. which list liquid oil as the first ingredient.
- b. which are the most resistant to rancidity.
- c. which have received the most hydrogenation.
- d. which are the most expensive products.

e   142   19. Triglycerides consist of:
- a. three fatty acids.
- b. *trans* fatty acids.
- c. glycerol.
- d. a and b
- e. a and c

c   145   20. Which of the following statements concerning lecithin is **not** true?
- a. It plays a key role in the structure of cell membranes.
- b. It is an emulsifier.
- c. It has the ability to lower blood cholesterol.
- d. It has no special ability to promote health.

d   150   21. DRI recommendations concerning intakes of fats include:
- a. consume up to 35% of calories as fat.
- b. keep saturated fat intake as low as possible.
- c. keep cholesterol intake at 100 mg.
- d. a and b
- e. b and c

c   159-160   22. Which of the following statements about *trans* fatty acids is **true**?
- a. They are made by the body.
- b. Their amounts are never listed on food labels.
- c. They arise when polyunsaturated oils are hydrogenated.
- d. They occur naturally in foods to a large extent.

e   161, 164-168   23. Which of the following food groups in the USDA Food Guide always contain fat?
                 a.   oils
                 b.   milk
                 c.   meats, poultry, fish, legumes, eggs and nuts
                 d.   a and b
                 e.   a and c

a   164   24. According to the USDA Food Guide, most adults should limit meat intake to 5-6 oz./day.
                 a.   true
                 b.   false

b   155-156   25. The best way to increase consumption of omega-3 fatty acids is to:
                 a.   increase intake of seed oils.
                 b.   consume 2–3 fish meals per week.
                 c.   limit intake of polyunsaturated fats.
                 d.   take fish oil in supplements.

a   164   26. Pork loin is an example of a lean cut of meat from which the fat can be trimmed.
                 a.   true
                 b.   false

d   162-163   27. Characteristics of the artificial fat olestra include:
                 a.   it passes through the digestive tract unabsorbed.
                 b.   it is fortified with vitamin E.
                 c.   it has no undesirable side effects.
                 d.   a and b
                 e.   b and c

c   151   28. An atherogenic diet is characterized by all of the following **except**:
                 a.   high in saturated fats.
                 b.   low in vegetables and fruits.
                 c.   low in *trans* fats.
                 d.   low in whole grains and legumes.

b   150-151   29. Which of the following is **not** a desirable blood lipid value?
                 a.   low total cholesterol
                 b.   high LDL
                 c.   high HDL
                 d.   low blood triglycerides

a   165   30. Some ground turkey and chicken products in which the skin is ground in are much higher in fats than lean beef.
                 a.   true
                 b.   false

Application Level Items

e   159   31. You see BHA listed in the ingredient list on a food product label. This is an example of:
                 a.   an additive.
                 b.   an emulsifier.
                 c.   an antioxidant.
                 d.   a and b
                 e.   a and c

c   143-4,165-6   32. You are talking with someone who is trying to decrease his intake of saturated and *trans* fat. Which of the following items would you recommend as a coffee whitener?
- a.   cream
- b.   non-dairy creamer
- c.   skim milk
- d.   half and half

e   143-144   33. Recent recommendations suggest that we consume monounsaturated fats in the place of saturated fat. Which of the following items would achieve this goal?
- a.   canola oil
- b.   safflower oil
- c.   olive oil
- d.   a and b
- e.   a and c

a   144, 160   34. You are trying to teach someone how to select an appropriate margarine to protect against heart disease. Therefore, you would tell the person to:
- a.   choose one that lists liquid oil as the first ingredient.
- b.   choose one that contains palm oil.
- c.   choose one that is labeled "vegetable oil."
- d.   choose one that is sold in a stick.

b   142   35. Approximately what percent calories from fat would be provided by a bowl of soup containing 200 calories and 99 calories from fat?
- a.   44%
- b.   50%
- c.   67%
- d.   72%

e   151-153   36. In an effort to lower LDL you would tell someone to:
- a.   use olive oil in the place of saturated fat.
- b.   use vegetable shortening in the place of lard.
- c.   use corn oil in the place of vegetable shortening.
- d.   a and b
- e.   a and c

d   151-153   37. People should not make efforts to reduce their intakes of food cholesterol very stringently because:
- a.   cholesterol is too widespread in all foods and it would result in a monotonous diet.
- b.   cholesterol-containing foods have a minimal effect on blood cholesterol in most people.
- c.   cholesterol-containing foods are nutritious and should not be eliminated from the diet.
- d.   b and c
- e.   a and b

e   148   38. Which of the following supports the statement that "you can get fatter on fat calories than on the same number of carbohydrate calories"?
- a.   To be stored as fat, glucose must undergo many chemical conversions in the body and each requires energy.
- b.   Compared to glucose, fat requires fewer chemical conversions in the body.
- c.   The body spends less energy assimilating carbohydrate than assimilating fat.
- d.   a and c
- e.   a and b

c   151   39. A 26-year-old male works in a high stress sales position. He has a family history of premature heart disease and he is physically inactive. How many risk factors for CVD does he have?

- a.   1
- b.   2
- c.   3
- d.   4

a   161   40. All of the following provide about 5 grams of pure fat **except:**

- a.   2 tablespoons sour cream.
- b.   1 teaspoon oil.
- c.   1 tablespoon salad dressing.
- d.   1 ½ teaspoons margarine.

c   145   41. Which of the following fats is the most saturated?

- a.   safflower oil
- b.   chicken fat
- c.   lard
- d.   coconut oil

b   145-146   42. All of the following statements concerning cholesterol are true **except:**

- a.   it is a part of every cell.
- b.   it is an essential nutrient.
- c.   it is important in the structure of brain and nerve cells.
- d.   it can be made by the body.

c   146-147   43. Which of the following statements best describes individuals who have had their gallbladder removed?

- a.   The liver stops producing bile.
- b.   They cannot digest food.
- c.   They must reduce their fat intake.
- d.   Bile is not delivered into the small intestine.

e   160   44. Which of the following words on an ingredient list would alert you to the presence of *trans* fatty acids in the product?

- a.   hydrogenated vegetable oil
- b.   liquid corn oil
- c.   shortening
- d.   a and b
- e.   a and c

Controversy Five – High-Fat Foods: Which to Choose for Good Health?

d   173   45. All of the following problems are associated with low-fat diets **except:**

- a.   they are difficult to maintain over time.
- b.   they are not necessarily low-calorie diets.
- c.   they may exclude nutritious foods.
- d.   they result in nutrient deficiencies.

a   173-174   46. The Mediterranean diet includes an eating style famous for supporting the health of the heart while including foods high in fat.

- a.   true
- b.   false

e   174   47. Overall, the diets of the Mediterranean people are:
  a.   low in saturated fat.
  b.   high in animal protein.
  c.   high in complex carbohydrates and fiber.
  d.   a and b
  e.   a and c

d   177   48. The Mediterranean Diet Pyramid classifies legumes as:
  a.   meats.
  b.   starches.
  c.   vegetables.
  d.   a separate category along with nuts.

d   174   49. Nutrient characteristics of nuts that may lower heart disease risk include:
  a.   they are high in dietary fiber.
  b.   they contain vitamin E, an antioxidant.
  c.   they are low in total fat.
  d.   a and b
  e.   a and c

b   175   50. The best source of EPA and DHA in the diet is:
  a.   nuts.
  b.   fish.
  c.   margarine.
  d.   olive oil.

Essay Questions

158-160   51. Describe the process of hydrogenation used to prevent spoilage of oils containing unsaturated fatty acids and discuss the advantages and disadvantages of this process.

157   52. Discuss arguments you would use in trying to convince someone to not take fish oil supplements.

159-160   53. What are *trans* fatty acids and what is their role in the promotion of heart disease?

149-151   54. Differentiate between LDL and HDL and explain why elevated LDL concentrations in the blood are a sign of high heart attack risk.

162-164   55. Describe olestra's side effects and discuss its potential impact on nutrition status.

140-141   56. Describe the useful functions of fats in the body.

145   57. Define the term emulsification and describe how the process of emulsification is used by food processors.

173-177   58. Compare and contrast the Mediterranean Diet Pyramid and the USDA Food Guide recommendations.

Ans.	Page	Comprehension Level Items

1. Which of the following is found in protein, as compared to carbohydrate and fat?
   a. carbon
   b. hydrogen
   c. nitrogen
   d. oxygen

   (Ans. c, Page 180)

2. Which of the following accounts for the differences between different amino acids?
   a. the amine group
   b. the side chain
   c. the acid group
   d. a and b
   e. b and c

   (Ans. b, Page 180)

3. How many amino acids are considered to be essential amino acids?
   a. 5
   b. 7
   c. 9
   d. 13

   (Ans. c, Page 181)

4. A _____ bond is formed between the amine group end of one amino acid and the acid group end of the next amino acid in a protein.
   a. peptide
   b. amino acid
   c. denatured
   d. sulfur

   (Ans. a, Page 181)

5. Which of the following is a protein catalyst which acts on other substances to change them chemically?
   a. hormone
   b. antibody
   c. catalyst
   d. enzyme

   (Ans. d, Page 182)

6. The sequences of amino acids that make up a protein molecule are specified by:
   a. age.
   b. sex.
   c. heredity.
   d. the diet.

   (Ans. c, Page 183)

7. All of the following cause denaturation of proteins **except:**
   a. bases.
   b. alcohol.
   c. heat.
   d. light.
   e. salts of heavy metals.

   (Ans. d, Page 184)

a 183   8. Sickle-cell disease is an example of an inherited mistake in the amino acid sequence.
     a.   true
     b.   false

b 184   9. For the majority of exercisers, adding excess protein or amino acid supplements to an adequate diet will stimulate muscle building.
     a.   true
     b.   false

a 193   10. When a person ingests a large dose of any single amino acid, absorption of others of its type may be limited.
     a.   true
     b.   false

b 191   11. When amino acids are degraded for energy, their amine groups are stripped off and used elsewhere or incorporated by the liver into:
     a.   bile.
     b.   urea.
     c.   glucose.
     d.   urine.

e 191   12. If amino acids are oversupplied:
     a.   the body stores them until they are needed.
     b.   the body removes and excretes their amine groups.
     c.   the body converts amino acid residues to glycogen or fat.
     d.   a and b
     e.   b and c

b 184   13. The stomach lining is protected from the very strong acid of the stomach by:
     a.   enzymes.
     b.   a coat of mucus.
     c.   saliva.
     d.   antibodies.

b 184   14. Some foods are so high in acid that they are capable of making the acid in the stomach even stronger.
     a.   true
     b.   false

a 199-200   15. Starvation always incurs wasting of lean body tissue as well as loss of fat.
     a.   true
     b.   false

a 191   16. If needed, protein can help to maintain a steady blood glucose level and so serve the glucose need of the brain.
     a.   true
     b.   false

d   192

17. Amino acids are wasted (not used to build protein or nitrogen-containing compounds) whenever there is:

    1. not enough energy from carbohydrate and fat.
    2. low-quality protein.
    3. too much protein.
    4. high-quality protein.

    a.   1 and 3
    b.   2 and 4
    c.   1, 3, and 4
    d.   1, 2, and 3

d   194-195

18. All of the following are needed for the body to synthesize protein **except:**
    a.   adequate carbohydrate and fat.
    b.   an adequate total amount of protein.
    c.   all essential amino acids in the proper amounts.
    d.   amino acid supplements.

b   194

19. Which of the following provides amino acids which are best absorbed by the body?
    a.   legumes
    b.   animal proteins
    c.   grains
    d.   vegetables

d   196

20. Of the following foods, which has the highest PDCAAS score?
    a.   chick peas
    b.   soybean protein
    c.   kidney beans
    d.   tuna

e   196

21. PDCAAS takes into account:
    a.   the digestibility of a protein.
    b.   the proportions of amino acids in a food.
    c.   how well the protein supports weight gain.
    d.   a and c
    e.   a and b

c   196

22. The DRI for protein depends on:
    a.   height.
    b.   weight.
    c.   body size.
    d.   sex.

b   196

23. The DRI Committee recommends _____ percent of total calories as the minimum amount of protein.
    a.   5
    b.   10
    c.   15
    d.   20

a   197

24. Negative nitrogen balance occurs in:
    a.   a surgery patient.
    b.   growing children.
    c.   pregnant women.
    d.   lactating women.

b   196   25. The DRI for protein for healthy adults is _____ grams per kilogram of body weight.
- a.   0.5
- b.   0.8
- c.   1.0
- d.   1.5

c   197   26. In making recommendations for protein intake, the committee on DRI took into consideration that the protein in a normal diet would be:
- a.   primarily from animal sources.
- b.   primarily from plant sources.
- c.   a combination of animal and plant sources.
- d.   used with 100% efficiency by everyone.

c   199   27. The calorie-deficiency disease is known as:
- a.   protein-calorie malnutrition.
- b.   kwashiorkor.
- c.   marasmus.
- d.   protein-energy malnutrition.

a   198   28. PEM is the world's most widespread form of malnutrition.
- a.   true
- b.   false

d   200   29. Which of the following is **not** a characteristic of children with kwashiorkor?
- a.   They retain some of their stores of body fat.
- b.   They accumulate fat in their livers.
- c.   They develop edema.
- d.   They look like skin and bones.

a   201   30. Which of the following is **not** associated with an excess of protein?
- a.   enlarged livers in humans
- b.   enlarged kidneys in animals
- c.   worsening of existing kidney problems
- d.   high-fat foods that contribute to obesity

e   202   31. Which of the following groups of the USDA Food Guide contribute(s) an abundance of high-quality protein?
- a.   vegetable
- b.   milk
- c.   meat
- d.   a and b
- e.   b and c

e   202   32. An overemphasis on protein-rich foods can lead to:
- a.   a low intake of iron.
- b.   a low intake of folate.
- c.   a low intake of vitamin C.
- d.   a and b
- e.   b and c

a   202   33. The more animal protein you eat, the higher your intake of _____.
- a.   vitamin B_{12}
- b.   vitamin A
- c.   folate
- d.   vitamin C

a   195   34. The strategy of combining two incomplete plant protein sources so that the amino acids in one food make up for those lacking in the other food is called:
- a.   mutual supplementation.
- b.   complementation.
- c.   simultaneous augmentation.
- d.   a and b
- e.   b and c

a   202   35. Most people in the U.S. would find it next to impossible not to meet their protein requirements.
- a.   true
- b.   false

a   180-181   36. The body normally makes tyrosine from the essential amino acid:
- a.   phenylalanine.
- b.   leucine.
- c.   valine.
- d.   lysine.

b   194   37. Which of the following cooking methods would you use to increase the digestibility of protein?
- a.   frying
- b.   stewing
- c.   grilling
- d.   baking

c   204   38. The heavy use of soy products in place of meat can inhibit _____ absorption.
- a.   calcium
- b.   folate
- c.   iron
- d.   vitamin C

d   199   39. A child with marasmus would exhibit all of the following symptoms **except:**
- a.   severe weight loss.
- b.   dry, thin and wrinkled skin.
- c.   apathy.
- d.   edema.

a   202-203   40. Which of the following food groups does **not** provide protein?
- a.   fruits
- b.   grains
- c.   vegetables
- d.   milk, yogurt and cheese

d   184   41. For athletes, the path to bigger muscles includes
- a.   vigorous physical training.
- b.   well-timed meals.
- c.   excess protein consumption.
- d.   a and b
- e.   b and c

b   186   42. Amino acid supplements are easy to digest and can relieve the digestive system from overworking.
- a.   true
- b.   false

a 188   43. Each of the millions of the body's red blood cells lives for only three or four months and must be replaced, which requires protein. This is an example of how protein is used for:
- a.   supporting growth and maintenance.
- b.   building enzymes, hormones, and other compounds.
- c.   building antibodies.
- d.   maintaining fluid and electrolyte balance.

Application Level Items

e 184   44. Why should eggs be cooked, rather than eaten raw?
- a.   Raw egg proteins bind the mineral iron.
- b.   Raw egg proteins speed up protein digestion.
- c.   Raw egg proteins bind the B vitamin biotin.
- d.   b and c
- e.   a and c

a 184   45. Why is milk used as a first-aid remedy for someone who has swallowed a heavy-metal poison?
- a.   The poison acts on the protein in the milk rather than on the protein of the gastrointestinal tract.
- b.   Milk will cause the person to vomit and expel the poison.
- c.   Milk will provide calcium which serves to render the poison unharmful.
- d.   a and b
- e.   b and c

e 184   46. Your friend states that she avoids acid foods like tomatoes and orange juice because they give her an acid stomach. How would you respond to this statement?
- a.   Highly acidic foods do increase the acidity of the stomach.
- b.   No food is acidic enough to make the stomach acid stronger.
- c.   The stomach is supposed to be acidic to do its job.
- d.   a and b
- e.   b and c

b 204   47. Your friend is a vegetarian who consumes large quantities of soy products in the place of meat. From a nutrition perspective, your friend is at risk of developing _____ deficiency.
- a.   vitamin C
- b.   iron
- c.   folate
- d.   calcium

e 191   48. An athlete consumes large amounts of meat in an effort to build extra muscle tissue. This practice does not work because:
- a.   the body has no place to store extra amino acids.
- b.   the body will dismantle its tissue proteins in this situation.
- c.   the body converts amino acid residues to fuel or stores them as fat.
- d.   a and b
- e.   a and c

a 196   49. Which of the following statements is/are true?
- a.   Athletes need slightly more protein than other healthy adults.
- b.   Athletes should consume protein supplements to build muscle.
- c.   Dieters should take protein supplements to spare body protein.
- d.   a and b
- e.   b and c

c   189, 200   50. A child suffering from protein deficiency has edema. This is an example of protein's role in:

        a.   supporting growth and maintenance.
        b.   building enzymes and hormones.
        c.   maintaining fluid and electrolyte balance.
        d.   maintaining acid-base balance.

d   196   51. Which of the following would have the lowest protein DRI?

        a.   a 28-year-old pregnant woman
        b.   a 6-year-old child
        c.   a 40-year-old male
        d.   a 34-year-old woman

c   196-197   52. What is the DRI for protein for a 40-year-old male who is 6'4" tall and weighs 180 pounds?

        a.   34 grams
        b.   49 grams
        c.   65 grams
        d.   144 grams

a   195-196   53. Examples of complementary protein combinations include all of the following **except:**

        a.   pasta with tomato sauce.
        b.   rice and black-eyed peas.
        c.   broccoli with walnuts.
        d.   peanut butter and jelly on whole-wheat bread.

Controversy Six – Vegetarian and Meat-Containing Diets: What are the Benefits and Pitfalls?

e   212   54. To ensure adequate intakes of vitamin B_{12}, vitamin D, and calcium, vegans need to:

        a.   select fortified foods.
        b.   use complete meal supplements.
        c.   use supplements daily.
        d.   a and b
        e.   a and c

a   207   55. Sound nutrition authorities acknowledge that well-chosen vegetarian diets are consistent with good health and can meet nutrient needs.

        a.   true
        b.   false

e   207, 208   56. Compared to meat eaters, vegetarians tend to have:

        a.   higher death rates from heart disease.
        b.   healthier body weights.
        c.   lower blood pressure.
        d.   a and b
        e.   b and c

a   209   57. The growth of well-fed vegetarian children is similar to that of their meat-eating peers.

        a.   true
        b.   false

b   208   58. Vegetarians have significantly higher rates of certain cancers than the general population.
             a.   true
             b.   false

d   210   59. Poorly-planned vegetarian diets typically lack all of the following **except:**
             a.   calcium.
             b.   vitamin B_{12}.
             c.   zinc.
             d.   folate.

Essay Questions

189-190   60. Explain how proteins help to regulate the quantity of fluids in the compartments of the body to maintain fluid and electrolyte balance.

193   61. Why would you advise someone to not take amino acid supplements?

199-200   62. Describe and differentiate between the causes and symptoms of marasmus and kwashiorkor.

191   63. Describe what happens when amino acids are oversupplied in the diet.

201-202   64. Discuss the risks associated with overconsumption of protein.

194   65. Describe factors that influence the digestibility of protein.

202, 204   66. Describe the advantages and limitations of consuming legumes as meat alternates.

208   67. Why do vegetarians have lower blood pressure than nonvegetarians?

208-209   68. Describe the relationship between vegetarian diets and risks of colon cancer.

Chapter 7 - The Vitamins

Ans.	Page	Comprehension Level Items

d   214   1. By definition, a vitamin is all of the following **except:**
- a. an organic compound.
- b. indispensable to body function.
- c. needed in minute amounts.
- d. a non-essential nutrient.

a   214   2. A compound in food that can be converted into an active vitamin inside the body is known as a(an):
- a. precursor.
- b. antivitamin.
- c. coenzyme.
- d. enzyme.

c   215   3. Any disease that produces _____ malabsorption can bring about deficiencies of vitamins A, D, E, and K.
- a. carbohydrate
- b. protein
- c. fat
- d. a and b
- e. b and c

e   228   4. True statements concerning the water-soluble vitamins include:
- a. They are stored in body tissues to a large extent.
- b. They are easily excreted in the urine.
- c. They can be leached out of foods by cooking in water.
- d. a and b
- e. b and c

c   215, 228   5. All of the following are fat-soluble vitamins **except:**
- a. A.
- b. D.
- c. C.
- d. K.

e   215   6. Vitamin A plays an important role in:
- a. maintenance of body linings.
- b. blood clotting.
- c. reproduction.
- d. a and b
- e. a and c

a   215   7. The active form of vitamin A stored in the liver is:
- a. retinol.
- b. bright orange.
- c. yellow.
- d. beta carotene.

c   218   8. Healthy people can eat vitamin A-rich foods in large amounts without risking toxicity, with the possible exception of:
a.   eggs.
b.   cheese.
c.   liver.
d.   fortified breakfast cereals.

d   217   9. Symptoms of vitamin A deficiency include:
a.   reduced food intake.
b.   blindness.
c.   joint pain.
d.   a and b
e.   a and c

d   219   10. All of the following foods contain active vitamin A **except:**
a.   liver.
b.   fish oils.
c.   milk.
d.   french fries.

d   220   11. Foods rich in beta carotene include:
a.   broccoli.
b.   sweet potatoes.
c.   beets.
d.   a and b
e.   b and c

a   219   12. The amount of vitamin A a person needs is proportional to:
a.   body weight.
b.   sex.
c.   age.
d.   season of the year.

b   219   13. To be assured of an adequate intake of vitamin A, a man needs a daily average of about _____ micrograms.
a.   700
b.   900
c.   1200
d.   1500

a   222   14. The vitamin D deficiency disease in adults is known as:
a.   osteomalacia.
b.   pellagra.
c.   rickets.
d.   macular degeneration.

d   222   15. Which of the following is the most potentially toxic of all vitamins?
a.   A
b.   E
c.   K
d.   D

a	222	16. Osteomalacia most often occurs in:

16. Osteomalacia most often occurs in:
    a. women with low calcium intake and little exposure to the sun who have repeated pregnancies and periods of lactation.
    b. children breastfed for an exceptionally long time.
    c. children with little exposure to the sun.
    d. men with low calcium intakes.

b   223

17. All of the following are significant food sources of vitamin D **except:**
    a. salmon.
    b. cereal.
    c. shrimp.
    d. fortified milk.

d   223

18. The recommended intake for vitamin D is _____ micrograms per day for adults over 70.
    a. 5
    b. 8
    c. 10
    d. 15

c   224

19. Vitamin E serves as:
    a. a precursor.
    b. a vitamin antagonist.
    c. an antioxidant.
    d. an antivitamin.

a   224-225

20. In which of the following situations would a vitamin E deficiency be least likely?
    a. someone who eats a diet high in fat
    b. someone who uses fat replacers as the only source of fat
    c. someone who consumes a low-fat diet composed largely of convenience foods
    d. someone with a disease condition that causes malabsorption of fat

c   226

21. As people consume more polyunsaturated oil their need for vitamin _____ rises.
    a. A
    b. D
    c. E
    d. K

b   227

22. A non-food source from which vitamin K can be obtained is:
    a. sunlight.
    b. intestinal bacteria.
    c. antibiotics.
    d. a and b
    e. b and c

c   227

23. The only animal food source which is rich in vitamin K is:
    a. milk.
    b. eggs.
    c. liver.
    d. fish.

c   233

24. The B vitamins act as part of:
    a. anticoagulants.
    b. antibodies.
    c. coenzymes.
    d. intrinsic factors.

b   242   25. The amount of _____ people need is proportional to protein intake.
  a.   niacin
  b.   vitamin B_6
  c.   folacin
  d.   vitamin B_{12}

d   235   26. The thiamin deficiency disease is known as:
  a.   pellagra.
  b.   osteomalacia.
  c.   scurvy.
  d.   beriberi.

b   236   27. Pellagra is a _____ deficiency disease.
  a.   vitamin C
  b.   niacin
  c.   thiamin
  d.   vitamin B_{12}

c   238   28. Which of the following B vitamins is especially important for women of childbearing age to prevent neural tube defects?
  a.   vitamin B_6
  b.   biotin
  c.   folate
  d.   vitamin B_{12}

a   241   29. An uninformed strict vegetarian is at special risk for _____ deficiency.
  a.   vitamin B_{12}
  b.   folate
  c.   vitamin B_6
  d.   niacin

d   229-230   30. Which of the following is **not** one of the functions of vitamin C?
  a.   protects against infections
  b.   produces and maintains collagen
  c.   promotes the absorption of iron
  d.   maintains bone density

a   230   31. In the U.S. scurvy is seldom seen today **except** in:
  a.   people addicted to alcohol.
  b.   young women.
  c.   vegetarians.
  d.   breastfed infants.

c   231   32. The DRI recommendation for vitamin C for women is _____ milligrams per day.
  a.   45
  b.   60
  c.   75
  d.   90

d   230-231   33. Which of the following should avoid vitamin C supplements?
  a.   people with kidney disorders
  b.   people with too much iron in their blood
  c.   people with colds
  d.   a and b
  e.   b and c

c   232   34. All of the following are good food sources of vitamin C **except:**
   a.   citrus fruits.
   b.   strawberries.
   c.   milk.
   d.   broccoli.

a   241   35. This vitamin aids in the conversion of tryptophan to niacin:
   a.   vitamin B_6.
   b.   vitamin C.
   c.   folate.
   d.   vitamin B_{12}.

b   220   36. Population studies suggest that people whose diets lack foods rich in beta-carotene have a higher incidence of:
   a.   rickets.
   b.   macular degeneration.
   c.   anemia.
   d.   osteomalacia.

e   224   37. Fortified plant sources of vitamin D available in the United States include:
   a.   yogurt.
   b.   margarine.
   c.   cereals.
   d.   a and b
   e.   b and c

c   226   38. Someone consuming a diet comprised mostly of processed, fast, deep-fried and convenience foods should be concerned about getting an adequate amount of vitamin:
   a.   A.
   b.   D.
   c.   E.
   d.   K.

d   228   39. Characteristics of water-soluble vitamins include all of the following **except**:
   a.   seldom reach toxic levels.
   b.   are easily absorbed and excreted.
   c.   dissolve in water.
   d.   are stored extensively in tissues.

b   239   40. The best natural sources of folate include:
   a.   cereals.
   b.   raw spinach.
   c.   cooked strawberries.
   d.   a and b
   e.   b and c

a   220   41. A higher incidence of macular degeneration is found in people whose diets lack foods rich in:
   a.   beta-carotene.
   b.   vitamin C.
   c.   vitamin E.
   d.   retinol.

d   226

42. About 20% of the vitamin E people consume comes from
   a.   vegetable oils and products made from them.
   b.   fruits and vegetables.
   c.   meats, fish, poultry, and eggs.
   d.   a and b
   e.   b and c

b   227

43. The main function of vitamin K is:
   a.   to act as an antioxidant in cell membranes.
   b.   to help synthesize proteins that help clot the blood.
   c.   to influence body functions through its regulation of the genes.
   d.   to help synthesize key bone proteins.

e   232

44. To derive the maximum amount of vitamin C from vegetables you would:
   a.   cut them into small pieces.
   b.   cook for short periods of time.
   c.   consume promptly after purchasing.
   d.   a and b
   e.   b and c

d   229-231

45. Which of the following statements regarding vitamin C is/are true?
   a.   It helps to protect against infection.
   b.   It helps in iron absorption.
   c.   It prevents the common cold.
   d.   a and b
   e.   b and c

Application Level Items

b   215

46. You advise your grandmother against using mineral oil as a laxative because:
   a.   the body cannot absorb it.
   b.   it may result in loss of the fat-soluble vitamins through excretion.
   c.   it may lead to toxic levels of the fat-soluble vitamins.
   d.   it is not an effective laxative.

c   215

47. If someone did not meet the recommended intakes for the fat-soluble vitamins one day, you would tell him to:
   a.   increase his consumption of foods rich in fat-soluble vitamins.
   b.   supplement his diet with a vitamin-mineral supplement.
   c.   not be concerned as long as the diet as a whole provides average amounts that approximate the recommended intakes.
   d.   try to consume more fats and oils to get the needed nutrients.

a   219-220

48. You eat frequently at fast food restaurants. In order to improve the nutritional quality and vitamin A content of a typical fast food meal you would:
   a.   order a salad with cheese and carrots.
   b.   order a large serving of fries.
   c.   drink a milkshake.
   d.   order a cheeseburger.

d	222	49. You have a friend who has very little exposure to the sun and she consumes very few calcium-rich foods. In addition, she has a 2-year-old child and 3-month-old twins. Your friend is at very high risk for developing: a. pellagra. b. rickets. c. beriberi. d. osteomalacia.
c	222-223	50. Which of the following would be able to make sufficient amounts of vitamin D without having to eat foods containing the vitamin? a. someone who goes to a tanning booth twice a week b. someone who works in an office with windows across an entire wall c. someone who wears light weight clothing and takes a walk outdoors d. someone with dark skin who takes a 15-minute walk each day
b	225	51. You have a friend who eats a lot of convenience foods and uses only diet margarine and diet salad dressings as sources of fat in her diet. You tell your friend that she is at risk for developing _____ deficiency. a. vitamin A b. vitamin E c. vitamin K d. vitamin D
d	226	52. Which of the following would provide the highest amount of vitamin E? a. whole milk b. a pork chop c. a fried chicken leg d. wheat germ oil
c	235	53. Which of the following groups would **not** be at risk for developing a thiamin deficiency? a. people who are addicted to alcohol b. people who consume polished rice as a food staple c. people who consume enough calories of whole foods d. a and b e. b and c
b	236-237	54. Which of the following would be most likely to develop pellagra? a. a person who consumes a mixed diet of meat and plant sources b. a person who does not consume meats and eats corn as the dietary staple c. a person who is a vegetarian but consumes milk d. a and b e. b and c

Controversy Seven: Vitamin Supplements: Who Benefits?

d	261	55. You recommend that your friend **not** take stress formula vitamin C supplements because: a. vitamin C is not involved in the release of the stress hormones from the adrenal gland. b. stress formula supplements are more expensive than other types of vitamin C supplements. c. the form of vitamin C in the supplements is not readily absorbed and utilized by the body. d. the amount of vitamin C used during stress can easily be obtained from generous servings of fruits and vegetables.

e   258   56. Antioxidant nutrients that actively scavenge and quench free radicals in the body include:
            a.   vitamin E.
            b.   riboflavin.
            c.   vitamin C.
            d.   a and b
            e.   a and c

a   259   57. Populations with high intakes of vegetables and fruits rich in antioxidant nutrients have
            low rates of:
            a.   cancer.
            b.   heart disease.
            c.   hypertension.
            d.   osteoporosis.

a   259   58. So far no convincing evidence exists indicating benefits from antioxidant supplements in
            well-nourished people.
            a.   true
            b.   false

e   260-261   59. The USP symbol on the label of a vitamin supplement means that:
            a.   it contains the ingredients as listed on the label.
            b.   it has been tested for effectiveness.
            c.   it will dissolve in the digestive tract.
            d.   a and b
            e.   a and c

a   261   60. A plant lacking a mineral or failing to make a needed vitamin dies before it can bear food
            for human consumption.
            a.   true
            b.   false

Essay Questions

215, 220   61. Differentiate between retinol and beta carotene and explain what retinol activity
            equivalents are.

221-223   62. Why are dark-skinned children who live in smoggy northern cities likely to develop
            rickets?

224-225   63. Identify specific diseases associated with vitamin E deficiency and describe why they
            have this effect.

215, 228   64. Compare and contrast the characteristics of the water-soluble vitamins and the fat-soluble
            vitamins.

238-239   65. Describe the rationale for the DRI Committee's recommendations for folate for women
            of childbearing age. What action has FDA taken to increase the folate content of the diets
            of this population group?

243   66. Describe how the B vitamins are related to heart disease.

260-261   67. Describe the major factors you would consider in choosing an appropriate multinutrient
            supplement.

256-258   68. Explain the labeling requirements that apply to supplements based on the Dietary
            Supplement Health and Education Act.

Chapter 8 - Water and Minerals

Ans.	Page	**Comprehension Level Items**

c   265

1. Which of the following makes up about 60 percent of the body's weight?
    - a. major minerals
    - b. protein
    - c. water
    - d. trace minerals

d   267

2. Water intake is governed by:
    - a. thirst.
    - b. sodium intake.
    - c. satiety.
    - d. a and c
    - e. b and c

e   268

3. Hard water has high concentrations of:
    - a. sodium.
    - b. calcium.
    - c. magnesium.
    - d. a and b
    - e. b and c

d   267

4. Water excretion is regulated by the:
    - a. brain.
    - b. kidneys.
    - c. stomach.
    - d. a and b
    - e. b and c

c   265

5. Which of the following is **not** characteristic of water?
    - a. Its molecules resist being crowed together.
    - b. It dissolves amino acids, glucose, and minerals.
    - c. It is a universal solvent.
    - d. It acts as a lubricant around joints.

d   265

6. Water assists in:
    - a. temperature regulation.
    - b. shock protection.
    - c. acid-base regulation.
    - d. a and b
    - e. b and c

a   266-267

7. Anyone who eats a meal high in salt can temporarily increase the body's water content.
    - a. true
    - b. false

c   267

8. The first sign of dehydration is:
    - a. headache.
    - b. confusion.
    - c. thirst.
    - d. fatigue.

d   273   9. Which of the following help prevent changes in the acid-base balance of body fluids?
   a.   proteins
   b.   vitamins
   c.   mineral salts
   d.   a and c
   e.   b and c

d   275   10. A person's absorption of calcium varies based on:
   a.   age.
   b.   vitamin D status.
   c.   gender.
   d.   a and b
   e.   b and c

c   293-294   11. Which of the following stabilizes bones and makes teeth resistant to decay?
   a.   cadmium
   b.   chloride
   c.   fluoride
   d.   mercury

a   273   12. Which of the following is the most abundant mineral in the body?
   a.   calcium
   b.   phosphorus
   c.   sodium
   d.   iron

b   274-275   13. Major roles of calcium in the body's fluids include all of the following **except:**
   a.   regulates the transport of ions across cell membranes.
   b.   helps maintain normal blood glucose.
   c.   is essential for the clotting of blood.
   d.   is essential for muscle contraction.

b   275   14. After about 25 years of age, regardless of calcium intake, bones begin to lose density.
   a.   true
   b.   false

d   275   15. Infants and children absorb about _____ percent of ingested calcium.
   a.   10
   b.   30
   c.   50
   d.   60

c   276   16. For women and men in the 19- to 50-year-old range, the calcium DRI is _____ milligrams.
   a.   600
   b.   800
   c.   1000
   d.   1200

c   299   17. The best way to obtain the calcium you need is to:
   a.   consume more spinach, rhubarb, and Swiss chard.
   b.   eat more cottage cheese and frozen yogurt.
   c.   consume more milk, cheese, and yogurt.
   d.   consume more cream cheese, butter, and cream.

c   279   18. The chief ion used to maintain the volume of fluid outside cells is:
                   a.   potassium.
                   b.   chloride.
                   c.   sodium.
                   d.   calcium.

a   279   19. Asian people may consume the equivalent of 30 to 40 grams of salt per day because of
                   their use of soy sauce and MSG.
                   a.   true
                   b.   false

b   279   20. A deficiency of sodium is not harmful.
                   a.   true
                   b.   false

d   279   21. Adults in the United States consume an average of _____ milligrams per day of
                   sodium.
                   a.   500
                   b.   1200
                   c.   2400
                   d.   3300

d   281   22. The more processed a food:
                   a.   the more sodium it contains.
                   b.   the less potassium it contains.
                   c.   the less sodium it contains.
                   d.   a and b
                   e.   b and c

d   281   23. Which of the following is the principal positively charged ion inside body cells?
                   a.   calcium
                   b.   sodium
                   c.   magnesium
                   d.   potassium

b   284, 298 24. Sulfate is adequate in a diet that contains sufficient:
                   a.   fat.
                   b.   protein.
                   c.   carbohydrate.
                   d.   vitamins.

c   277   25. Over half of the body's magnesium is stored in the:
                   a.   teeth.
                   b.   liver.
                   c.   bones.
                   d.   kidneys.

a   284   26. The principal food source of chloride is:
                   a.   salt.
                   b.   animal products.
                   c.   plants.
                   d.   grains.

b   284   27. Which of the following must be available for thyroxine to be synthesized?
- a.   iron
- b.   iodine
- c.   zinc
- d.   fluoride

d   290   28. Which of the following impairs iron absorption?
- a.   tea
- b.   phytates
- c.   vitamin C
- d.   a and b
- e.   b and c

e   289   29. The DRI iron intake recommendation is 8 mg/day for:
- a.   women 19-50 years of age.
- b.   men.
- c.   women 51 years or older.
- d.   a and b
- e.   b and c

c   292   30. Which of the following foods provides the least amount of available zinc?
- a.   meats
- b.   poultry
- c.   legumes
- d.   shellfish

a   277   31. The best source of phosphorus is:
- a.   animal protein.
- b.   fruit.
- c.   vegetable protein.
- d.   grain products.

c   268   32. Which of the following foods has the lowest percentage of water?
- a.   Chinese cabbage
- b.   fresh apple
- c.   margarine
- d.   lean steak

b   269   33. Which of the following agencies is responsible for ensuring that public water systems meet minimum standards for protection of public health?
- a.   Food and Drug Administration
- b.   Environmental Protection Agency
- c.   Food Safety and Inspection Service
- d.   World Health Organization

d   271   34. Which of the following would you look for on the label of bottled water to signify safety?
- a.   a symbol of the Food and Drug Administration
- b.   a source indicating the water is from a spring in your state
- c.   a label with the terms "mountain spring water"
- d.   a trademark of the International Bottled Water Association

a   293-294   35. Which of the following minerals hardens and stabilizes the crystals of teeth and makes the enamel resistant to decay?
   a. fluoride
   b. phosphorus
   c. calcium
   d. chloride

b   292   36. Low blood selenium correlates with development of:
   a. breast cancer.
   b. prostate cancer.
   c. stomach cancer.
   d. colon cancer.

a   294   37. Chromium works closely with:
   a. insulin.
   b. collagen.
   c. hemoglobin.
   d. enzymes.

d   272, 294   38. Which of the following best describes the fluoride content of bottled water?
   a. high
   b. low
   c. moderate
   d. unpredictable

a   300   39. The bioavailability of calcium in calcium-fortified orange juice is comparable to that of milk.
   a. true
   b. false

c   292   40. Which of the following foods provides the highest amount of zinc?
   a. legumes
   b. whole-grain bread
   c. shellfish
   d. spinach

Application Level Items

b   265   41. Which characteristic of water is represented by its ability to act as a lubricant?
   a. ability to act as solvent
   b. incompressibility
   c. heat-holding capacity
   d. a and b
   e. b and c

c   268-269   42. A friend informs you that she is planning to purchase a water softener. Which of the following statements would be most appropriate for you to make to your friend?
   a. Soft water makes more bubbles with less soap than hard water and is more desirable.
   b. Hard water leaves a ring in the tub and a gray residue in the wash which are undesirable.
   c. Soft water appears to aggravate hypertension and heart disease which is undesirable.
   d. Soft water has higher concentrations of calcium and magnesium than hard water which is desirable.

c   268   43. How much water and fluid beverages (in cups) should a man consume each day, under moderate environmental conditions and given a normal diet?
- a.   6
- b.   9
- c.   13
- d.   15

a   275   44. Which of the following groups absorb the least amount of calcium?
- a.   adults
- b.   children
- c.   infants
- d.   pregnant women

c   275   45. Which of the following statements is true?
- a.   People develop their peak bone during the first four decades of life.
- b.   The skeleton no longer adds to bone density after 30 years of age.
- c.   The bones begin to lose density after 40 years of age regardless of calcium intake.
- d.   People do not need calcium throughout life.

a   299   46. Which of the following would be the best selection to provide good sources of calcium in the diet?
- a.   milk, yogurt, and ice milk
- b.   kefir, butter, and cottage cheese
- c.   buttermilk, cream cheese, and almonds
- d.   cheese, cream, and broccoli

b   279   47. How much sodium is consumed by a person who eats two grams of salt?
- a.   400 mg
- b.   800 mg
- c.   1000 mg
- d.   1200 mg

c   291   48. You are working with a child in a health clinic who has growth retardation, impaired immunity, and a poor appetite. This child is most likely experiencing _____ deficiency.
- a.   iron
- b.   chromium
- c.   zinc
- d.   magnesium

d   286-287   49. Your best friend complains that she is tired all of the time and has a problem concentrating. In addition, she likes to chew ice. Which of the following is your friend likely to have?
- a.   potassium deficiency
- b.   zinc deficiency
- c.   magnesium deficiency
- d.   iron deficiency

b   289-290   50. Which of the following would you consume with a food source of iron in order to facilitate iron absorption?
- a.   tea and a soy protein hamburger
- b.   tomato and meat, fish or poultry
- c.   coffee and wheat bran muffins
- d.   calcium supplement and whole wheat bread

Controversy Eight – Osteoporosis: Can Lifestyle Choices Reduce the Risks?

d   304-305   51. Which of the following ethnic groups has the highest bone density?
- a. Asians
- b. Hispanics
- c. Mexican Americans
- d. Africans

e   305   52. After age 65, calcium absorption declines because:
- a. older people tend to lose lean body mass.
- b. aging skin is less efficient at making vitamin D.
- c. some of the hormones change and accelerate bone mineral withdrawal.
- d. a and b
- e. b and c

a   305   53. Whether a person develops osteoporosis seems to depend partly on heredity and partly on the environment, including nutrition.
- a. true
- b. false

b   306   54. Osteoporosis is most often associated with:
- a. heavier body weights.
- b. underweight.
- c. higher body fatness.
- d. exercise.

a   309-310   55. Authorities recommend foods as a source of calcium in preference to calcium supplements.
- a. true
- b. false

Essay Questions:

267   56. Identify and explain factors involved in governing water intake and water excretion.

268-269   57. Would you discourage someone from purchasing a water softener? Provide a rationale for your answer.

275   58. What is peak bone mass and when is it developed?

279   59. Explain the rationale for the following statement: "The way to keep body salt and water weight under control is to control salt intake and drink more, not less, water."

286   60. Differentiate between iron deficiency and iron-deficiency anemia and describe the causes and symptoms of the latter.

280   61. Describe the characteristics of DASH (Dietary Approaches to Stop Hypertension).

289   62. Explain the rationale for the argument against high-level iron fortification in foods.

308-310   63. Why do nutrition authorities recommend foods as the source of calcium rather than supplements?

306-307   64. Describe what is known about the relationship between a high-protein diet and bone loss.

280   65. Describe the relationship between salt and blood pressure in salt sensitive people. Who is at greatest risk for being salt sensitive?

Chapter 9 - Energy Balance and Healthy Body Weight

Ans.	Page	Comprehension Level Items

b   312   1. Which of the following is **not** a health risk associated with deficient body fat?
   a.   increased risk during hospitalization
   b.   increased risk of developing hypertension
   c.   increased risk for individuals fighting a wasting disease
   d.   increased chance of death from cancer

d   313   2. Excess body fatness is associated with an increased risk of:
   a.   some cancers.
   b.   gallbladder disease.
   c.   diverticular disease.
   d.   a and b
   e.   b and c

d   326   3. The theory that the body tends to maintain a certain weight by means of its own internal controls is referred to as the _____ theory.
   a.   enzyme theory
   b.   fat cell theory
   c.   thermogenesis
   d.   set-point

b   323   4. The psychological desire to eat is referred to as:
   a.   satiety.
   b.   appetite.
   c.   hunger.
   d.   obesity.

d   324   5. All of the following are involved in signaling satiation **except**:
   a.   the stomach.
   b.   small intestine.
   c.   brain's hypothalamus.
   d.   the heart.

b   313   6. Women in their reproductive years are likely to carry more intraabdominal fat than are women past menopause.
   a.   true
   b.   false

a   314   7. Waist circumference reflects the degree of _____ in proportion to body fatness.
   a.   visceral fatness
   b.   central obesity
   c.   subcutaneous fat
   d.   total body fatness

b   314   8. A body mass index of 25.0 to 29.9 in an adult indicates:
   a.   normal weight.
   b.   overweight.
   c.   underweight.
   d.   obesity.

b 313 9. Excess fat around the _____ represents a greater risk to health than excess fat elsewhere on the body.
   a. hips
   b. central abdominal area
   c. shoulders
   d. chest

d 322 10. A woman of normal weight may have, on the average, _____ percent of the body weight as fat.
   a. 5
   b. 10
   c. 15
   d. 20

c 316 11. One pound of body fat is equal to _____ calories.
   a. 2500
   b. 3000
   c. 3500
   d. 4000

a 316 12. Taller people need proportionately more energy than shorter people to balance their energy budgets.
   a. true
   b. false

d 317 13. Which of the following are true statements about basal metabolism?
   a. It supports the work that goes on all the time.
   b. It is directly controlled by the hormone thyroxine.
   c. It accounts for the smallest component of the average person's daily energy expenditure.
   d. a and b
   e. b and c

d 332 14. The three kinds of energy nutrients can be stored in the body as:
   a. glycogen.
   b. water.
   c. fat.
   d. a and c
   e. a and b

a 332-333 15. Which of the following is **not** a true statement?
   a. Carbohydrate from food is especially easy for the body to store as fat.
   b. Protein is stored in the body in response to exercise.
   c. Alcohol delivers calories and encourages fat storage.
   d. Any food can make you fat it you eat enough of it.

a 330 16. In early food deprivation, the nervous system cannot use _____ as fuel.
   a. fat
   b. glucose
   c. protein
   d. carbohydrate

d   330

17. A healthy person starting with average body fat can live totally deprived of food for as long as six to eight weeks due to:
   a.   acidosis.
   b.   thermogenesis.
   c.   metabolism.
   d.   ketosis.

c   332

18. Any low-calorie diet is accompanied by:
   a.   lean tissue loss.
   b.   ketosis.
   c.   loss of appetite.
   d.   fast weight loss.

b   317

19. All of the following factors are associated with a higher basal metabolic rate **except:**
   a.   stress.
   b.   starvation.
   c.   fever.
   d.   youth.

c   335

20. Nutrition authorities agree that the staple foods of high-protein, low-carbohydrate diets clearly raise the risk for:
   a.   osteoporosis.
   b.   kidney disease.
   c.   heart and artery disease.
   d.   cancer.

a   332

21. The DRI Committee recommends at least 130 grams of carbohydrate a day.
   a.   true
   b.   false

e   347

22. Successful weight maintainers:
   a.   exercise regularly.
   b.   wait until severely hungry to eat.
   c.   keep track of food intake and exercise habits.
   d.   a and b
   e.   a and c

d   316

23. Older people generally need less energy than younger people due to:
   a.   slowed basal metabolic rate.
   b.   declines in lean body mass.
   c.   decreases in height.
   d.   a and b
   e.   a and c

b   329, 342

24. Physical activity must be long and arduous to achieve fat loss.
   a.   true
   b.   false

a   329

25. Quick, large changes in weight are most likely the result of all of the following **except:**
   a.   changes in fat.
   b.   changes in body fluid content.
   c.   changes in bone minerals.
   d.   changes in lean tissues such as muscles.

b   318   26. Eating certain foods can elevate the basal metabolic rate, and thus promote weight loss.
            a.   true
            b.   false

b   317   27. About _____ percent of a meal's energy value is used up in stepped-up metabolism
            in the five or so hours following each meal.
            a.   1-5
            b.   5-10
            c.   10-15
            d.   15-20

e   347   28. A person who diets without exercising:
            a.   will never lose body weight.
            b.   often becomes trapped in weight cycling.
            c.   will be more susceptible to regaining weight lost.
            d.   a and b
            e.   b and c

a   314   29. Which of the following has replaced weight-for-height tables in clinical settings?
            a.   BMI
            b.   fatfold test
            c.   bioelectrical impedance
            d.   dual energy X-ray absorptiometry

d   343-344 30. A person trying to gain weight should:
            a.   participate in physical activity.
            b.   eat more frequently.
            c.   eat faster.
            d.   a and b
            e.   a and c

b   345   31. Which of the following strategies would be appropriate for an obese individual with a
            BMI of 40 or above who is healthy?
            a.   an herbal supplement
            b.   surgery such as a gastric bypass
            c.   liposuction or lipectomy
            d.   an ephedrine-containing dietary supplement

a   327   32. For someone with at least one obese parent, the chance of becoming obese is estimated to
            be between 40 and 70 percent.
            a.   true
            b.   false

e   320   33. Body Mass Index is unsuitable for use with:
            a.   adolescents.
            b.   athletes.
            c.   pregnant women.
            d.   a and b
            e.   b and c

d   322   34. Hunger makes itself known roughly ___ hours after eating.
            a.   1-2
            b.   2-3
            c.   3-5
            d.   4-6

d   325   35. Which of the following types of foods sustain satiety longer?
                  a.   high in fiber
                  b.   high in protein
                  c.   high in sugar
                  d.   a and b
                  e.   b and c

d   335   36. The Committee on DRI links high-protein diets with increased risk of:
                  a.   cancer.
                  b.   osteoporosis.
                  c.   malnutrition.
                  d.   a and b
                  e.   b and c

c   345   37. Complications immediately following obesity surgery often include all of the following **except:**
                  a.   dehydration.
                  b.   infection.
                  c.   vitamin and mineral deficiencies.
                  d.   nausea.

b   343   38. Exercise can remove the fat from any one particular area of the body.
                  a.   true
                  b.   false

d   342   39. Health professionals advise people to engage in these types of activities for weight loss:
                  a.   low to moderate intensity.
                  b.   long duration.
                  c.   high intensity.
                  d.   a and b
                  e.   b and c

a   320   40. Waist circumference indicates visceral fatness, and above a certain girth, disease risks rise, even when BMI values are normal.
                  a.   true
                  b.   false

Application Level Items

d   316   41. John routinely consumes 7,000 calories per day in excess of his energy expenditure. How much body fat would John store per day as a result of this practice?
                  a.   ½ pound
                  b.   1 pound
                  c.   1 ½ pounds
                  d.   2 pounds

e   320   42. You are weighing a team of football players and according to the BMI values they appear to be obese. Which of the following would you most likely conclude?
                  a.   The majority of them are probably obese and should make efforts to lose weight.
                  b.   Their muscle weight is probably responsible for the elevated scale weights.
                  c.   Their bones may be well mineralized, which contributes to their weights.
                  d.   a and b
                  e.   b and c

a	343-344	43. James is trying to gain weight. Which of the following would you suggest to help James with his goal?

a   343-344   43. James is trying to gain weight. Which of the following would you suggest to help James with his goal?
        a.   Choose milkshakes instead of milk.
        b.   Drink black coffee.
        c.   Drink beverages with meals.
        d.   Skip dessert.

e   313-314   44. Mary has a waist circumference of 38 inches. Based on this information you conclude that:
        a.   she develops fat centrally.
        b.   she has a large amount of subcutaneous fat.
        c.   she is at an increased risk for disease.
        d.   a and b
        e.   a and c

d   314, 327   45. Johnnie's father is 5' 11" tall and weighs 165 pounds, while his mother weighs 145 pounds and is 5' 2" tall. Johnnie's chances of becoming obese are at least ___ percent.
        a.   10
        b.   20
        c.   30
        d.   40

c   327-328   46. Susie has been overweight for many years. She tends to eat when she is not really hungry and eats more food when she is angry or depressed. Which of the following could explain Susie's problem of overweight?
        a.   enzyme theory
        b.   set-point theory
        c.   external cues
        d.   fat cell number theory

b   317   47. Paul is a 19-year-old athlete who is 6' tall and weighs 178 pounds; Rick is a 40-year-old salesman who weighs 165 pounds and is 5' 7" tall. Who would have the higher basal metabolic rate?
        a.   Rick
        b.   Paul

b   338   48. Donna weighs 160 pounds. How many grams of fat should Donna consume in order to meet the DRI recommendation, if she consumes 1600 calories a day?
        a.   20-45
        b.   35-62
        c.   45-70
        d.   > 70

Controversy Nine: The Perils of Eating Disorders

d   353   49. Characteristics of victims of anorexia nervosa include:
        a.   they come from middle- or-upper class families.
        b.   they tend to be perfectionists.
        c.   they are unfamiliar with the calorie content of foods.
        d.   a and b
        e.   b and c

c	353	50. Central to the diagnosis of anorexia nervosa is:

50. Central to the diagnosis of anorexia nervosa is:
   a.   fear of gaining weight.
   b.   amenorrhea.
   c.   a distorted body image.
   d.   weight loss.

a   354   51. Bulimia is more prevalent than anorexia nervosa and is more common in women than men.
   a.   true
   b.   false

b   355   52. Characteristics of bulimia include all of the following **except:**
   a.   the victim is close to her ideal body weight.
   b.   the victim is unaware that her behavior is abnormal.
   c.   the victim's weight fluctuates 10 pounds or so over a few weeks.
   d.   the victim binges and purges.

a   356   53. Society plays a role in eating disorders because they are known only in developed nations and they become more prevalent as wealth increases and food becomes plentiful.
   a.   true
   b.   false

Essay Questions

317-318   54. How would you respond to an advertisement for a weight loss diet that claims that eating certain foods can elevate the BMR and thus promote weight loss? How can someone change his or her BMR?

313-314   55. Identify three groups of people who are more prone to develop central obesity. Why is fat that collects in the central abdominal area of the body especially dangerous?

318-320   56. Describe the advantages and drawbacks of using body mass index for assessing obesity.

325-326   57. Briefly describe the metabolic theories for the cause of obesity.

330-332   58. Define ketone bodies and describe what happens when the body goes into ketosis.

343-344   59. Describe strategies that can help someone effectively gain body weight.

335   60. Explain the potential hazards that can accompany high-protein, low-carbohydrate diets.

351-352   61. Describe what is meant by the female athlete triad.

354   62. Describe the appropriate treatment for someone with anorexia nervosa.

Chapter 10 – Nutrients, Physical Activity, and the Body's Responses

Ans.	Page	Comprehension Level Items

c   362

1. Which of the following is **not** a component of fitness?
   a. flexibility
   b. muscle strength
   c. balance
   d. muscle endurance
   e. cardiorespiratory endurance

d   362

2. Which of the following enhances flexibility?
   a. weight training
   b. aerobic activity
   c. calisthenics
   d. stretching

e   362

3. Muscles respond to the overload of exercise by gaining:
   a. strength.
   b. fat.
   c. size.
   d. a and b
   e. a and c

c   364

4. Active people can have resting pulse rates of _____ beats per minute or lower.
   a. 30
   b. 40
   c. 50
   d. 70

e   364

5. Characteristics of cardiorespiratory endurance include:
   a. increased cardiac output and oxygen delivery.
   b. reduced blood pressure.
   c. increased resting pulse.
   d. a and c
   e. a and b

c   364

6. In the early minutes of an activity, _____ provides the majority of energy the muscles use to go into action.
   a. fat
   b. liver glycogen
   c. muscle glycogen
   d. protein

a   364

7. As physical activity continues, which of the following flow into the bloodstream to signal the liver and fat cells to liberate their stored energy nutrients?
   a. epinephrine
   b. thyroxine
   c. lactic acid
   d. a and b
   e. a and c

b	367	8. Anaerobic glucose breakdown produces fragments of glucose molecules that accumulate in the tissues and blood called: a. urea. b. lactic acid. c. uric acid. d. amino acid.

b   367   8. Anaerobic glucose breakdown produces fragments of glucose molecules that accumulate in the tissues and blood called:
   a.   urea.
   b.   lactic acid.
   c.   uric acid.
   d.   amino acid.

d   368   9. A person who continues exercising moderately for longer than _____ minutes begins to use less glucose and more fat for fuel.
   a.   5
   b.   10
   c.   15
   d.   20

a   375   10. Iron-deficiency anemia impairs physical performance because iron helps deliver the muscles' oxygen.
   a.   true
   b.   false

e   369   11. Which of the following is (are) included in a safe plan for carbohydrate loading?
   a.   severely restricting carbohydrate intake before the competition
   b.   gradually cutting back on activity during the week before competition
   c.   eating a high-carbohydrate diet during the three days before competition
   d.   a and b
   e.   b and c

b   366-369   12. This factor does **not** influence how much glucose a person uses during physical activity:
   a.   carbohydrate intake.
   b.   age of the person exercising.
   c.   duration of the activity.
   d.   degree of training of the muscles.

d   368   13. Strategies which help endurance athletes maintain their blood glucose concentrations for as long as they can include:
   a.   eating a high-carbohydrate diet regularly.
   b.   taking in glucose during endurance activity.
   c.   consuming fat and protein before the event.
   d.   a and b
   e.   b and c

d   376   14. The first symptom of dehydration is:
   a.   hypoglycemic.
   b.   heavy breathing.
   c.   heat stroke.
   d.   fatigue.

b   376   15. The body's need for _____ far surpasses that for any other nutrient.
   a.   fat
   b.   water
   c.   carbohydrate
   d.   protein

c	377	16. During exercise the optimal beverage for replacing fluids is:
		    a. a beverage that supplies glucose.
		    b. fruit juice.
		    c. cool water.
		    d. a salt solution.

a	372	17. Most athletes probably need somewhat more protein than do sedentary people.
		    a. true
		    b. false

c	376	18. The digestive system can absorb about one _____ of fluid an hour.
		    a. cup
		    b. pint
		    c. quart
		    d. gallon

d	380	19. For athletic performance the diet should consist of all of the following **except**:
		    a. nutrient-dense foods.
		    b. foods moderate in fat.
		    c. foods high in carbohydrates.
		    d. foods high in protein.

a	360	20. People who regularly engage in physical activity live longer on average than those who are physically inactive.
		    a. true
		    b. false

c	382	21. Any meal should be finished at least _____ hours before an athletic competition.
		    a. 1 or 2
		    b. 2 or 3
		    c. 3 or 4
		    d. 4 or 5

a	379	22. Moderate use of caffeine by athletes:
		    a. may assist performance.
		    b. slows down reactions.
		    c. depletes glycogen stores.
		    d. has no adverse effects.

e	379	23. Which of the following should **not** be used by athletes?
		    a. sports beverages
		    b. carbonated beverages
		    c. alcohol
		    d. a and b
		    e. b and c

d	363	24. Progressive weight training is **not** associated with:
		    a. increased muscle strength.
		    b. management of cardiovascular disease.
		    c. greater bone density.
		    d. reduced lean body tissue.

b   372   25. Protein contributes an average of about _____ percent of the total fuel used during activity and during rest.
- a.   5
- b.   10
- c.   15
- d.   20

d   371   26. The length of time the basal metabolic rate remains elevated after exercise depends on:
- a.   the duration of the activity.
- b.   the intensity of the activity.
- c.   the composition of the diet.
- d.   a and b
- e.   b and c

b   373   27. The American Dietetic Association recommends _____ gram(s) protein per kilogram of body weight each day for an endurance athlete.
- a.   0.8 - 1.2
- b.   1.2 - 1.6
- c.   1.6 - 2.2
- d.   2.2 - 2.6

d   373   28. Which of the following nutrients is important for athletes because it is needed for the formation of collagen?
- a.   vitamin E
- b.   iron
- c.   thiamin
- d.   vitamin C

a   374   29. The most important antioxidant related to physical activity is:
- a.   vitamin E.
- b.   beta carotene.
- c.   vitamin C.
- d.   folate.

e   375   30. Sports anemia:
- a.   is a normal adaptation to endurance training.
- b.   requires treatment with iron supplements.
- c.   is temporary.
- d.   a and b
- e.   a and c

a   378   31. Sports drinks offer some advantages over water for athletes who:
- a.   need to replenish electrolytes.
- b.   are older.
- c.   exercise outside in cold weather.
- d.   a and b
- e.   b and c

b   368   32. Glycogen depletion occurs after about ___ hours of vigorous activity.
- a.   one
- b.   two
- c.   three
- d.   four

c	370	33. Sports nutrition experts recommend that endurance athletes consume ____ percent of their energy from fat. a. 5-10 b. 10-20 c. 20-30 d. 30-40
d	375	34. Which of the following are most prone to iron deficiency? a. female athletes b. endurance athletes c. power athletes d. a and b e. b and c
b	382	35. To consume an adequate amount of B vitamins, magnesium, and chromium an athlete should eat: a. meats. b. whole grains. c. leafy vegetables. d. milk.
a	363	36. To emphasize muscle endurance in weight training, you would combine less resistance (lighter weights) with more repetitions. a. true b. false
d	363	37. Weight training results in all of the following **except:** a. improved posture. b. muscle strength and endurance. c. prevention and management of chronic diseases. d. decreased bone density.
b	376	38. Active people do not need extra fluid in cold weather. a. true b. false
e	379	39. To prevent hyponatremia during prolonged events, athletes should: a. drink large amounts of water over the course of the event. b. favor sports drinks over water. c. eat pretzels in the last half of a long event. d. a and b e. b and c
c	382-383	40. Which of the following is an advantage of sports bars for athletes? a. They provide complete nutrition. b. They are inexpensive. c. They are easy to eat in the hours before competition. d. They are superior to homemade snacks.

Application Level Items

c 372 41. Which of the following athletes would use less protein for fuel during exercise?
   a. Joe, who consumes a protein-rich diet
   b. Charles, who consumes a fat-rich diet
   c. Gary, who consumes a carbohydrate-rich diet
   d. Rick, who consumes a diet rich in branched-chain amino acids

e 375 42. An athlete is in the early weeks of an aerobic training program and develops a decrease in hemoglobin concentration. Which of the following is true?
   a. The condition is called sports anemia.
   b. It probably reflects a low iron intake.
   c. It goes away by itself.
   d. a and b
   e. a and c

d 379 43. Carbonated beverages are not a good choice for meeting an athlete's fluid needs because they:
   a. do not enhance athletic performance.
   b. speed up the use of glycogen.
   c. have a potentially hazardous diuretic effect.
   d. make a person feel full quickly and may limit fluid intake.

a 374 44. An athlete takes vitamin and mineral supplements prior to competition because he believes they can enhance performance. How would you respond to this practice?
   a. The practice does not improve performance because there is not enough time for them to be combined with other appropriate parts so they can do their work.
   b. The practice has been supported by research and advocated by health care professionals.
   c. The practice is beneficial because athletes tend to be deficient in vitamins and minerals.
   d. The practice improves performance because the vitamin has time to combine with its other appropriate parts before competition.

d 377 45. A female athlete weighs 120 pounds before a race and 115 pounds after the race. How much fluid should she consume?
   a. 2 cups
   b. 5 cups
   c. 7 cups
   d. 10 cups

b 378-379 46. Your friend participates in strenuous world-class competition that lasts for four hours or more. Which of the following would you recommend to your friend?
   a. Suggest that he not worry about electrolyte losses.
   b. Suggest that he consume sports drinks and pretzels.
   c. Suggest that he take electrolyte or salt tablets.
   d. Suggest that he drink plain water.

d 379 47. Why would you tell someone **not** to drink alcohol before engaging in an athletic event?
   a. because it is a diuretic
   b. because it makes people nervous
   c. because it promotes excretion of vitamins such as thiamin
   d. a and c
   e. b and c

75

d	380	**48.** How many grams of carbohydrate would an athlete need to consume to ensure full glycogen and other nutrient stores and to meet energy needs if he consumes 2800 calories?
		   a. 140 grams
		   b. 202 grams
		   c. 350 grams
		   d. 490 grams

c	382	**49.** Which of the following would **not** be appropriate as part of a pregame meal?
		   a. toast and pineapple juice
		   b. pancakes with syrup
		   c. high-fiber cereal with low-fat milk
		   d. baked potato and orange juice

a	376	**50.** Which of the following is the best fluid for an athlete working out in a cold climate?
		   a. room temperature water
		   b. cold water
		   c. a sports drink
		   d. a sweat replacer

Controversy Ten – Ergogenic Aids: Breakthroughs, Gimmicks, or Dangers?

a	388	**51.** Which of the following statements regarding carnitine is true?
		   a. It is a nonessential nutrient.
		   b. It is a fat burner.
		   c. The more carnitine consumed, the more energy produced.
		   d. a and b
		   e. b and c

d	385	**52.** The term *ergogenic*:
		   a. implies that the product has special work-enhancing powers.
		   b. is associated with supplements claimed to benefit athletes.
		   c. implies that the product is safe to consume.
		   d. a and b
		   e. b and c

c	389	**53.** Muscle growth is stimulated by:
		   a. excess protein in the diet.
		   b. branched-chain amino acids.
		   c. physically demanding activity.
		   d. amino acid supplements.

e	389	**54.** Which of the following is (are) characteristics of candy bars and specialty drinks marketed to athletes?
		   a. They provide extra food energy.
		   b. They provide "complete" nutrition.
		   c. They can be useful as a pregame meal.
		   d. a and b
		   e. a and c

b	389	**55.** Which of the following is among the most dangerous and illegal ergogenic practices?
		   a. chromium picolinate
		   b. anabolic steroid hormones
		   c. creatine
		   d. DHEA and androstenedione

Essay Questions

363-364   56. Identify the characteristics and benefits of cardiorespiratory endurance.

382-383   57. Describe the composition and characteristics of an ideal pregame meal.

375   58. Why are vegetarian female athletes particularly vulnerable to iron deficiency?

375   59. Differentiate between the causes, characteristics, and treatment of iron-deficiency anemia and sports anemia.

369   60. Describe the appropriate procedure for carbohydrate loading.

360-361   61. Describe the health benefits from physical activity.

363   62. Describe the benefits of weight training.

387-388   63. Describe the potential benefits versus adverse effects of caffeine use among athletes.

389   64. Describe the side effects of taking steroid hormone drugs.

361   65. Explain how physical activity lowers the risk of cardiovascular disease.

Ans.	**Page**	**Comprehension Level Items**

b   394

1. Degenerative diseases are the only type of diseases that afflict people in developed countries.
   a.   true
   b.   false

a   396

2. A deficiency or toxicity of even a single nutrient can weaken the body's defenses considerably.
   a.   true
   b.   false

d   394, 396

3. Which of the following holds the key to maintaining the best possible immune system support?
   a.   nutrient supplements
   b.   herbal remedies
   c.   phytochemicals
   d.   adequate nutrition

c   396

4. Which of the following must be given careful attention when feeding the person with AIDS?
   a.   soft foods
   b.   small frequent snacks
   c.   food safety
   d.   Daily Food Guide recommendations

d   395-396

5. Effects of protein-energy malnutrition on the body's defense system include:
   a.   skin becomes thinner with less connective tissue.
   b.   antibody secretions and immune cell number are reduced.
   c.   immune system organs increase in size.
   d.   a and b
   e.   b and c

a   394

6. Degenerative diseases are often referred to as chronic diseases.
   a.   true
   b.   false

c   402

7. Which of the following would be considered a risk factor for CVD?
   a.   total blood cholesterol below 200 mg/dl
   b.   HDL higher than 60 mg/dl
   c.   LDL 160 mg/dl or higher
   d.   triglycerides less than 150 mg/dl

d   401-402

8. Which of the following is **not** one of the risk factors for CVD?
   a.   diabetes
   b.   hypertension
   c.   high blood LDL
   d.   high blood HDL

b   398   9. CVD is a man's disease.
             a.   true
             b.   false

d   401   10. In men, aging becomes a significant risk factor for heart disease at age:
             a.   30.
             b.   35.
             c.   40.
             d.   45.

a   405   11. Wherever dietary fat consists mostly of _____ fats and fish, fruits, and vegetables
             are eaten in abundance, blood cholesterol and the rate of death from heart disease are
             low.
             a.   unsaturated
             b.   saturated
             c.   *trans*
             d.   omega-6

d   406   12. According to the DRI Committee, the percentage of calories from fat in the diet should
             be no more than _____ percent.
             a.   20
             b.   25
             c.   30
             d.   35

e   422   13. The Canadian "Reach for It" and U.S. "5 a Day" programs encourage people to:
             a.   consume enough whole grains.
             b.   consume enough fruits.
             c.   consume enough vegetables.
             d.   a and b
             e.   b and c

a   401-402, 405   14. Which of the following is associated with a reduced risk of CVD?
             a.   high HDL
             b.   high total cholesterol
             c.   high LDL
             d.   high triglycerides

e   404, 407   15. Which of the following raise HDL concentration?
             a.   moderate alcohol intake
             b.   low cholesterol intake
             c.   physical activity
             d.   b and c
             e.   a and c

a   404   16. Thirty minutes of light, balanced exercise, performed at intervals throughout the day, can
             improve the odds against heart disease.
             a.   true
             b.   false

b   406   17. All of the following dietary factors are protective against CVD **except:**
             a.   omega-3 fatty acids.
             b.   insoluble fiber.
             c.   flaxseed.
             d.   nuts.

c   409   18. Resting blood pressure should ideally be _____ or lower.
- a.   100 over 70
- b.   110 over 75
- c.   120 over 80
- d.   140 over 90

e   409   19. Which of the following is(are) risk factors for the development of hypertension?
- a.   age
- b.   gender
- c.   genes
- d.   a and b
- e.   a and c

d   411   20. Salt sensitive individuals are likely to include:
- a.   African Americans.
- b.   those who are less than 50 years of age.
- c.   those who have diabetes.
- d.   a and c
- e.   b and c

d   412   21. Which of the following appear to help prevent and treat hypertension in certain populations?
- a.   magnesium
- b.   potassium
- c.   folate
- d.   a and b
- e.   b and c

e   418   22. Alcohol alone is associated with cancers of the:
- a.   mouth.
- b.   head and neck.
- c.   breast.
- d.   a and b
- e.   a and c

c   412   23. Individuals with hypertension being treated with diuretics should consume foods rich in:
- a.   calcium.
- b.   magnesium.
- c.   potassium.
- d.   folate.

a   413   24. Constituents in foods may be cancer causing, cancer promoting, or protective against cancer.
- a.   true
- b.   false

d   416   25. In general, studies of populations have suggested that low cancer rates correlate with:
- a.   high vegetable intakes.
- b.   high whole grain intakes.
- c.   high fat intakes.
- d.   a and b
- e.   b and c

a   417   26. Laboratory studies suggest that diets high in _____ seem to promote cancer.
- a. calories
- b. salt
- c. alcohol
- d. calcium

a   417   27. Excess calories from carbohydrates, protein, and fat all raise cancer rates.
- a. true
- b. false

d   420   28. Examples of cruciferous vegetables include:
- a. rutabaga.
- b. bok choy.
- c. green onions.
- d. a and b
- e. a and c

b   419   29. Which of the following nutrients plays a special role with respect to cervical and colon cancer?
- a. vitamin E
- b. folate
- c. beta-carotene
- d. vitamin C

d   420, 423   30. The best action to take to decrease your risk of cancer is to:
- a. limit foods that are grilled, smoked and charbroiled.
- b. consume a diet moderate in fat.
- c. take vitamin supplements.
- d. eat a wide variety of vegetables and fruits in generous quantities every day.

a   420   31. Which of the following may offer a protective effect against colon cancer?
- a. calcium
- b. potassium
- c. magnesium
- d. folate

c   405   32. The metabolic syndrome greatly increases a person's risk of developing:
- a. hypertension.
- b. cancer.
- c. CVD.
- d. AIDS.

e   404   33. To lower LDL cholesterol levels you would tell someone to:
- a. lose weight.
- b. consume a low-fat diet.
- c. increase physical activity.
- d. a and b
- e. a and c

a   406   34. In dietary recommendations to decrease the risk of CVD, *trans*-fatty acids are classified with this type of fat:
- a. saturated.
- b. polyunsaturated.
- c. unsaturated.
- d. monounsaturated.

c   411   35. To help prevent hypertension Americans should limit their sodium intake to _____ mg.
      a.   2000
      b.   2200
      c.   2300
      d.   2600

b   394   36. Dietary supplements can trigger extra immune power to fend off dangerous infections.
      a.   true
      b.   false

a   405   37. Metabolic syndrome approaches the power of high LDL cholesterol in raising the risk of CVD.
      a.   true
      b.   false

b   406   38. For people living in the United States and Canada, saturated fat in the diet should account for no more than _____ percent of calories.
      a.   5
      b.   10
      c.   20
      d.   30

d   405   39. An atherogenic diet is characterized as one:
      a.   high in saturated fats.
      b.   high in *trans* fats.
      c.   high in polyunsaturated fats.
      d.   a and b
      e.   b and c

a   417   40. The risk of cancer rises with BMI.
      a.   true
      b.   false

Application Level Items

c   396   41. You have a friend with AIDS and are trying to support his nutrition status. Which of the following would you do?
      a.   offer large, frequent meals
      b.   encourage consumption of megadoses of nutrient supplements
      c.   cook foods thoroughly and practice cleanliness
      d.   cook a lot of food in advance and leave it out for your friend

d   406   42. To help control blood cholesterol you would:
      a.   consume oats, barley, and legumes.
      b.   limit foods with *trans* fatty acids.
      c.   eliminate eggs from your diet.
      d.   a and b
      e.   b and c

e   406   43. To minimize risks of CVD you would:
      a.   choose more fruits and whole grains.
      b.   stir-fry all of your vegetables.
      c.   choose more fish and poultry.
      d.   a and b
      e.   a and c

b 402 44. All of the following are risk factors for CVD **except:**
  a. LDL cholesterol of 150 mg/dl.
  b. diastolic blood pressure of 80.
  c. HDL cholesterol of 25 mg/dl.
  d. blood cholesterol of 240 mg/dl.

d 423 45. Jack's physician has placed him on a diet recommended by the National Heart, Lung, and Blood Institute to control his blood cholesterol. In order to follow this plan Jack would:
  a. consume ≤ 200 mg cholesterol per day.
  b. consume 25-35% of calories as fat.
  c. consume 30% of calories as monounsaturated fats.
  d. a and b
  e. a and c

e 406-407 46. You are interested in controlling your risk of developing CVD. Which of the following would you do?
  a. consume high levels of complex carbohydrates and fiber
  b. substitute fish for red meat twice a week
  c. use margarine in the place of olive oil
  d. a and c
  e. a and b

b 409-410 47. Which of the following individuals is at highest risk for developing hypertension?
  a. Susie, a 30-year-old female who is slightly overweight
  b. Jack, a 40-year-old African American male whose parents had hypertension
  c. Jill, a 50-year -old female of Asian descent who consumes a diet relatively high in sodium
  d. Bill, a 45-year-old male of European descent who is a vegetarian

e 416-417 48. Dietary guidelines for cancer prevention include:
  a. controlling energy intake.
  b. increasing intake of salt-cured products.
  c. increasing intake of fruits and vegetables.
  d. a and b
  e. a and c

b 411 49. Jeff is a 54-year-old male who is 5' 6" tall, weighs 165 pounds, and has hypertension. The single most effective dietary measure Jeff can take is to:
  a. consume less sodium.
  b. reduce his weight.
  c. increase intake of potassium.
  d. consume adequate calcium.

e 418-420 50. To reduce your risks of developing cancer you would:
  a. reduce intake of saturated fat only.
  b. have a high fruit and vegetable intake.
  c. consume whole grains and other fiber-rich foods.
  d. a and b
  e. b and c

Controversy Eleven: The Obesity Epidemic—How Can We Gain Control?

e   426-427   51. An obesity promoting environment is one characterized by:
- a.   a sedentary lifestyle.
- b.   increased exposure to advertising.
- c.   consumption of high-energy foods.
- d.   a and b
- e.   a and c

c   429-430   52. Nutrition education has all but disappeared from the nation's classrooms due to:
- a.   ineffectiveness of nutrition education.
- b.   lack of preparation.
- c.   federal funding cuts.
- d.   lack of student interest.

c   426   53. The average person in the United States today consumes about _____ calories per day more than in 1970.
- a.   300
- b.   400
- c.   500
- d.   600

d   427   54. Today's meals are most often influenced by:
- a.   which foods are readily available.
- b.   which foods are easiest to prepare.
- c.   which foods are more nutritious.
- d.   a and b
- e.   b and c

a   428   55. The strategy of offering more food for even a little more money at each selling opportunity pays off in greater profits for food-related businesses.
- a.   true
- b.   false

Essay Questions

395-396   56. Describe the effects that protein-energy malnutrition has on the various immune-system organs and tissues.

397-398   57. How would you decide whether certain diet recommendations are especially important to you to decrease your risk of degenerative diseases?

405-408   58 Describe dietary and other strategies for reducing risk of CVD.

409   59. Explain how atherosclerosis can make hypertension worse.

405   60. Describe what is meant by the metabolic syndrome.

411   61. Explain what is meant by the term *salt sensitive* and describe the characteristics of people most prone to this condition.

416-421   62. Describe characteristics of diets that are thought to be protective against cancer.

428   63. Describe techniques that are used to sell foods and other products to youth.

429-430   64. Explain actions that the government can initiate to reverse obesity trends.

Chapter 12 - Food Safety and Food Techology

Ans	Page	Comprehension Level Items

c   434   1. Which of the following hazards in our food supply is of most concern according to the Food and Drug Administration?
    a.   natural toxins
    b.   food additives
    c.   microbial foodborne illness
    d.   environmental contaminants

a   434   2. The FDA has identified genetic modification of foods as the area of least concern in our food supply.
    a.   true
    b.   false

b   462   3. The agency charged with the responsibility of deciding what additives shall be in foods is the:
    a.   United States Department of Agriculture.
    b.   Food and Drug Administration.
    c.   Environmental Protection Agency.
    d.   Federal Trade Commission.

d   463   4. Which of the following statements is(are) true concerning the GRAS list?
    a.   It includes a list of additives believed to be safe.
    b.   It stands for generally recognized as safe.
    c.   It is not subject to revision as new facts become known.
    d.   a and b
    e.   a and c

a   462   5. Food additives used in the U.S. are strictly controlled and pose little cause for concern.
    a.   true
    b.   false

a   465   6. Only _____ synthetic color additives are still approved by the FDA for use in foods.
    a.   10
    b.   33
    c.   47
    d.   66

c   465   7. Which of the following additives are among the most intensively investigated of all additives?
    a.   flavor enhancers
    b.   antimicrobial agents
    c.   artificial colors
    d.   antioxidants

d	466	8. Which of the following is the largest single group of food additives?
		    a. antioxidants
		    b. coloring agents
		    c. antimicrobial agents
		    d. flavoring agents

e	466	9. Monosodium glutamate:
		    a. is used widely in Asian restaurants.
		    b. is an example of a flavor enhancer.
		    c. can be added to foods for infants.
		    d. a and c
		    e. a and b

d	464	10. Which of the following is(are) the best known and most widely used antimicrobial agents?
		    a. salt
		    b. nitrites
		    c. sugar
		    d. a and c
		    e. a and b

d	464	11. Nitrites are added to foods to:
		    a. enhance their flavor.
		    b. preserve their color.
		    c. improve their nutritive value.
		    d. a and b
		    e. a and c

d	464	12. Which of the following causes cancer in animals?
		    a. nitrites
		    b. sulfites
		    c. BHA
		    d. nitrosamines

a	465	13. Which of the following is **not** used as an antioxidant in foods?
		    a. vitamin A
		    b. vitamin E
		    c. sulfites
		    d. vitamin C

c	465	14. A person choosing a food that contains sulfites should not count on that food to provide a share of the daily need for:
		    a. niacin.
		    b. riboflavin.
		    c. thiamin.
		    d. vitamin C.

d	467	15. Nutrient additives are commonly found in:
		    a. breakfast cereals.
		    b. dairy products.
		    c. snack foods.
		    d. a and b
		    e. a and c

e   440   16. Which of the following should **not** be used to thaw frozen meats?
a.   refrigerator thawing
b.   defrosting at room temperature
c.   defrosting in a bath of warm water
d.   a and b
e.   b and c

b   456   17. Which of the following is(are) **not** intentionally used in or on foods?
a.   additives
b.   contaminants
c.   pesticides
d.   a and b
e.   b and c

d   460   18. A processing technique that preserves food by killing all microorganisms present in food and sealing out air is called:
a.   freezing.
b.   drying.
c.   extrusion.
d.   canning.

e   460   19. The canning process is based on:
a.   exposure to air.
b.   time.
c.   temperature.
d.   a and c
e.   b and c

b   460-461   20. Which of the following statements concerning thiamin is **not** true?
a.   Acid stabilizes thiamin.
b.   It is sensitive to light.
c.   Thiamin is lost during canning.
d.   Heat rapidly destroys thiamin.

a   460   21. Fat-soluble vitamins and minerals are not affected much by canning.
a.   true
b.   false

e   462   22. Sulfite additives added during the drying of fruits results in:
a.   prevention of browning.
b.   destruction of vitamin C.
c.   destruction of thiamin.
d.   a and b
e.   a and c

d   461   23. Frozen foods' nutrient content is similar to that of:
a.   dried foods.
b.   canned foods.
c.   foods which have undergone extrusion.
d.   fresh foods.

c	461	24. Losses of _____ are especially likely during the freezing process.

     a.   riboflavin
     b.   thiamin
     c.   vitamin C
     d.   niacin

d   461

25. Results of drying foods include:
     a.   it eliminates microbial spoilage.
     b.   it reduces the weight and volume of foods.
     c.   it causes major nutrient losses.
     d.   a and b
     e.   a and c

e   462

26. Characteristics of foods which have undergone extrusion include:
     a.   they usually have had nutrients added to them.
     b.   they should be used as staple foods.
     c.   they have undergone considerable nutrient losses.
     d.   a and b
     e.   a and c

c   444

27. Which of the following is especially susceptible to bacterial contamination?
     a.   roast
     b.   steak
     c.   ground meat
     d.   chicken

b   447-448

28. Which of the following foods would you **not** choose for a picnic?
     a.   fresh fruits
     b.   mixed salad of chopped ingredients
     c.   breads and crackers
     d.   canned cheeses

e   446

29. Which of the following groups should avoid all uncooked or undercooked eggs?
     a.   the elderly
     b.   healthy adults
     c.   those who suffer immune dysfunction
     d.   a and b
     e.   a and c

c   446-447

30. To prevent serious illness from consuming raw oysters you would:
     a.   consume them with hot sauce.
     b.   drink whiskey with the oysters.
     c.   eat them fully cooked and not raw.
     d.   a and b
     e.   b and c

e   449

31. To avoid poisoning by toxins you would:
     a.   consume a variety of foods.
     b.   eat only "natural" foods.
     c.   eat all foods in moderation.
     d.   a and b
     e.   a and c

d	454	32. To reduce your intake of pesticide residue you would:
		    a. trim fat from meat.
		    b. discard the outer layers of cabbage.
		    c. bite into the peel of an orange.
		    d. a and b
		    e. b and c

d	440	33. After cooking, foods should be held at ____° F or higher until served.
		    a. 110
		    b. 120
		    c. 130
		    d. 140

b	447	34. All varieties of sushi are made from raw fish.
		    a. true
		    b. false

e	455	35. Which of the following has placed a ban on the use of bST for milk cows?
		    a. European Union
		    b. United States
		    c. Canada
		    d. a and b
		    e. a and c

c	460	36. Modified atmosphere packaged foods compare well to _____ foods in terms of nutrient quality.
		    a. frozen
		    b. dried
		    c. fresh
		    d. canned

a	465	37. BHT protects against cancer through an antioxidant effect similar to that of vitamin E.
		    a. true
		    b. false

b	467	38. Incidental food additives sometimes find their way into foods, and adverse effects are common.
		    a. true
		    b. false

Application Level Items

d	435	39. To be sure that your home-canned food does not contain the botulinum toxin you would:
		    a. follow proper canning techniques.
		    b. boil the canned food for 10 minutes.
		    c. test the soil in which the food was grown.
		    d. a and b
		    e. b and c

d	444-445	40. To prevent foodborne illness you would:
		    a. use a meat thermometer to roast a whole chicken.
		    b. cook hamburgers to well-done.
		    c. cook your roast in the microwave.
		    d. a and b
		    e. b and c

e   446   41. Billy loves to eat raw seafood and does so frequently. As a result, Billy runs the risk of suffering from:
a.   hepatitis.
b.   AIDS.
c.   worms.
d.   a and b
e.   a and c

d   448   42. Joe is planning a trip to Mexico and wants to practice food safety while traveling. You would tell Joe to:
a.   eat raw fruits.
b.   use lots of ice in beverages.
c.   use the local water supply.
d.   avoid salads.

b   461   43. Which of the following would lose the most riboflavin?
a.   low-acid foods
b.   glass-packed foods
c.   canned foods
d.   foods processed with acid

e   469-470   44. To minimize the loss of water-soluble vitamins from vegetables you would:
a.   microwave them.
b.   soak them in water.
c.   steam them over water.
d.   a and b
e.   a and c

d   461   45. Which of the following would be least likely to lose any vitamin C during the freezing process?
a.   peaches
b.   pineapples
c.   apples
d.   strawberries

b   462   46. Dried peaches which have been processed with sulfite additives would provide a good source of:
a.   thiamin.
b.   vitamin C.
c.   riboflavin.
d.   iron

e   469   47. To protect the vitamin content of fruits and vegetables, you would:
a.   keep them at room temperature.
b.   select vine ripened ones.
c.   chill immediately after picking.
d.   a and b
e.   b and c

a   465   48. You are interested in using a preservative which will prevent a food from undergoing changes in color and flavor caused by exposure to oxygen in the air. Which of the following would you use?
      a.   tocopherol
      b.   nitrites
      c.   tartrazine
      d.   salt

a   451   49. Properly irradiated food does not become radioactive.
      a.   true
      b.   false

d   451   50. Which of the following is (are) **not** required to bear a label stating that they have been irradiated?
      a.   spices mixed with processed foods
      b.   foods served in restaurants
      c.   fresh fruits
      d.   a and b
      e.   b and c

a   450   51. Several scientific and health organizations have concluded that irradiation of food is safe and can improve food safety in the United States and the world.
      a.   true
      b.   false

Controversy Twelve: Organic Foods and Genetically Modified Foods: What Are the Pros and Cons?

d   474   52. Among the successes of selective breeding is:
      a.   soybeans.
      b.   tomatoes.
      c.   potatoes.
      d.   corn.

e   473   53. Regulations for the production of certified organic foods specify that:
      a.   plant foods must be produced without the use of synthetic fertilizers and pesticides.
      b.   animals may be subjected to high-stress habitats that are unnatural to them.
      c.   they cannot use ingredients produced by irradiation and biotechnology.
      d.   a and b
      e.   a and c

b   474   54. Which of the following types of foods is (are) **not** required to be labeled as such?
      a.   irradiated
      b.   genetically modified
      c.   organic
      d.   a and b
      e.   b and c

a   473   55. The word *organic* on the label is no guarantee that a food is:
      a.   pesticide-free.
      b.   fertilized with manure or vegetable compost.
      c.   grown without hormones or antibiotics.
      d.   produced without genetic modification.

e   474   56. Those individuals purchasing organic foods are urged to:
- a.   buy unpastuerized juices.
- b.   wash raw produce vigorously.
- c.   cook the food properly.
- d.   a and b
- e.   b and c

Essay Questions

462-463   57. Describe the special procedure a manufacturer has to go through to get permission to use a new additive in food products.

442-443   58. Describe three methods of eliminating microbes on kitchen cutting boards and utensils and identify the advantages and disadvantages of each.

460-461   59. Contrast and compare the nutrient losses which occur with canning versus freezing.

446-447   60. Why is eating raw or lightly steamed seafood a risky business?

449   61. Can consumers concerned about food contamination eliminate all poisons from their diet by eating only "*natural*" foods? Why or why not? What would you recommend to avoid toxicities from natural food constituents?

469   62. Why is milk sold in cardboard or opaque plastic containers?

439   63. Describe the prevention method known as Hazard Analysis Critical Control Point (HACCP).

474-479   64. Outline the arguments in support of and in opposition to genetic engineering.

478-480   65. Describe the FDA's position on genetically modified foods.

446   66. Why are foodborne illnesses from raw produce increasing and becoming more troublesome?

Chapter 13 - Life Cycle Nutrition
Mother and Infant

<u>Ans</u>	<u>Page</u>	<u>**Comprehension Level Items**</u>

c | 482 | 1. Which of the following is the single most potent indicator of an infant's future health status?

    a.   mother's prepregnancy weight
    b.   mother's weight gain during pregnancy
    c.   infant's birthweight
    d.   mother's prepregnancy nutrition status

a | 482 | 2. A low-birthweight baby is nearly 40 times more likely to die in the first year of life than is a normal-weight baby.

    a.   true
    b.   false

d | 482 | 3. Which of the following is the major factor in low birthweight?

    a.   heredity
    b.   smoking
    c.   drug use during pregnancy
    d.   poor nutrition

a | 484 | 4. The two weeks following fertilization are considered to be a critical period developmentally for the zygote.

    a.   true
    b.   false

a | 483 | 5. Which of the following determines whether the mother is able to grow a healthy placenta?

    a.   the mother's prepregnancy nutrition
    b.   the mother's prepregnancy weight
    c.   whether or not the mother receives vitamin supplementation
    d.   a and b
    e.   b and c

c | 483 | 6. All of the following statements are true concerning the placenta **except:**

    a.   it is an active metabolic organ with many responsibilities.
    b.   it allows for the exchange of materials between baby and mother.
    c.   the fetus receives nutrients and carbon dioxide across the placenta.
    d.   the mother's blood picks up the baby's waste materials through the placenta and they are excreted.

e | 484 | 7. At eight weeks of development, the fetus is characterized by:

    a.   a beating heart.
    b.   fully formed facial features.
    c.   a fully formed digestive system.
    d.   a and b
    e.   a and c

93

c   482   8. The stage of human gestation from eight weeks after conception until birth of an infant is called a(an):
        a.   embryo.
        b.   zygote.
        c.   fetus.
        d.   ovum.

d   484   9. Early malnutrition in the mother affects the baby's:
        a.   heart.
        b.   brain.
        c.   lungs.
        d.   a and b
        e.   b and c

b   485   10. During the second trimester of pregnancy, a daily increase of _____ calories above the allowance for nonpregnant women is recommended.
        a.   2235
        b.   340
        c.   450
        d.   530

a   487   11. A pregnant woman needs about _____ grams of protein per day above prepregnancy needs.
        a.   25
        b.   30
        c.   35
        d.   40

a   487   12. All pregnant women need generous amounts of _____ to spare their protein and to provide energy.
        a.   carbohydrate
        b.   fat
        c.   protein
        d.   calories

a   487   13. During pregnancy, the recommended carbohydrate intake is between 135 and 175 grams per day.
        a.   true
        b.   false

e   488   14. The pregnant woman's greater need for folate is due to:
        a.   the great increase in her blood volume.
        b.   the increase in protein needs.
        c.   the rapid growth of the fetus.
        d.   a and b
        e.   a and c

c   488   15. Which of the following nutrients is related to the prevention of neural tube defects?
        a.   vitamin B_6
        b.   vitamin B_{12}
        c.   folate
        d.   zinc

b 489   16. Which of the following does **not** contain vitamin B_{12}?
           a.   meat
           b.   legumes
           c.   eggs
           d.   dairy products

e 490   17. Which of the following statements is(are) true concerning iron during pregnancy?
           a.   The body conserves iron even more than usual.
           b.   Absorption of iron decreases.
           c.   Iron supplements are needed.
           d.   a and b
           e.   a and c

a 489   18. Folate fortification has lowered the number of neural tube defects that occur each year.
           a.   true
           b.   false

a 489   19. The DRI recommendation for calcium intake is the same for non-pregnant and pregnant
               women in the same age group.
           a.   true
           b.   false

d 493   20. A woman who craves nonnutritious substances during pregnancy:
           a.   may have a nutrient-poor diet.
           b.   is experiencing pica.
           c.   is experiencing an adaptive behavior.
           d.   a and b
           e.   b and c

c 491   21. A pregnancy weight gain of _____ pounds is recommended for women who are at
               their appropriate weights.
           a.   13
           b.   15 - 25
           c.   25 - 35
           d.   28 - 40

b 491   22. The ideal pattern of weight gain is thought to be about _____ pounds total during
               the first three months of pregnancy.
           a.   2
           b.   3 ½
           c.   4
           d.   4 ½

a 492   23. Physical activity during pregnancy can improve fitness, facilitate labor, and reduce
               psychological stress.
           a.   true
           b.   false

c 493   24. A pregnant teenager with a body mass index in the normal range is encouraged to gain
               _____ pounds or so.
           a.   13
           b.   20
           c.   35
           d.   42

a   491   25. The weight that pregnant women put on is nearly all lean tissue.
           a.   true
           b.   false

a   491   26. A sudden, large weight gain during pregnancy is always a danger signal.
           a.   true
           b.   false

d   496-497   27. Which of the following should be avoided during pregnancy?
           a.   alcohol
           b.   dieting
           c.   caffeine consumption
           d.   a and b
           e.   b and c

a   499   28. All pregnant women should be assessed for gestational diabetes risk at their first prenatal examination.
           a.   true
           b.   false

c   499   29. Which of the following is **not** one of the key elements to help identify women with preeclampsia?
           a.   edema
           b.   hypertension
           c.   convulsions
           d.   protein in the urine

e   494   30. The nausea of morning sickness:
           a.   arises from hormonal changes of early pregnancy.
           b.   can be avoided.
           c.   can often be alleviated.
           d.   a and b
           e.   a and c

d   494   31. Constipation during pregnancy should be relieved by:
           a.   a high-fiber diet.
           b.   plentiful water intake.
           c.   the use of laxatives.
           d.   a and b
           e.   b and c

d   500   32. A nursing mother produces about _____ ounces of milk a day.
           a.   10
           b.   15
           c.   20
           d.   25

a   506   33. The composition of breast milk changes from early milk for the newborn to later milk to feed the older infant.
           a.   true
           b.   false

b   500   34. The effect of maternal nutritional deprivation during lactation is to:
       a.   reduce the quality of milk.
       b.   reduce the quantity of milk.
       c.   make breastfeeding impossible.
       d.   a and b
       e.   b and c

c   506   35. If the water supply is severely deficient in _____, both breastfed and formula-fed infants require supplementation after six months of age.
       a.   vitamin C
       b.   zinc
       c.   fluoride
       d.   iron

b   506   36. It is desirable to begin feeding the infant iron-fortified cereals by about _____ months.
       a.   three
       b.   six
       c.   nine
       d.   twelve

d   505   37. Characteristics of breast milk include:
       a.   its sodium content is low.
       b.   its protein is largely alpha-lactalbumin.
       c.   its vitamin C content is poor.
       d.   a and b
       e.   b and c

e   506   38. Characteristics of colostrum include the following:
       a.   it contains antibodies from the mother's blood.
       b.   it contains white cells from the mother's blood.
       c.   it may transmit a bacterial infection to the infant if the mother has one.
       d.   a and c
       e.   a and b

d   506   39. Most babies are born with enough _____ to last about half a year.
       a.   calcium
       b.   fluoride
       c.   vitamin D
       d.   iron

b   509   40. The addition of foods to a baby's diet should be governed by all of the following considerations **except:**
       a.   the baby's nutrient needs.
       b.   how often the baby cries.
       c.   the baby's physical readiness to handle different forms of foods.
       d.   the need to detect and control allergic reactions.

a   491   41. For normal weight women, the ideal pattern of weight gain after the first trimester is one pound per week.
       a.   true
       b.   false

d	487	42. All of the following are recommended for vegetarian women who are pregnant **except:**
		    a. legumes.
		    b. tofu.
		    c. whole grains.
		    d. high-protein supplements.

e	489	43. To obtain the folate that can reduce the risk of neural tube defects, a woman who is capable of becoming pregnant should:
		    a. eat folate-fortified foods.
		    b. take a daily supplement containing 800 micrograms of folic acid.
		    c. eat folate-rich foods.
		    d. a and b
		    e. a and c

d	489	44. These minerals are in great demand during pregnancy because they are involved in building the skeleton:
		    a. phosphorus.
		    b. magnesium.
		    c. zinc.
		    d. a and b
		    e. b and c

a	482	45. A low-birthweight baby is defined as one who weighs less than 5 ½ pounds.
		    a. true
		    b. false

b	487	46. A pregnant woman should strive to meet her DRI for _____ by increasing intakes of milk, cheese, yogurt and other foods rich in this mineral, or by taking a 600 mg supplement daily.
		    a. sodium
		    b. calcium
		    c. iodine
		    d. potassium

d	489	47. Fortified food sources of folate include all of the following **except:**
		    a. pasta.
		    b. bread.
		    c. bagels.
		    d. orange juice.

e	494	48. To prevent heartburn during pregnancy you would recommend:
		    a. eating less frequently.
		    b. relaxing and eating slowly.
		    c. avoiding greasy and spicy foods.
		    d. a and b
		    e. b and c

a	495-496	49. The FDA and EPA advise pregnant women to eat up to 12 ounces a week of a variety of safer fish and shellfish such as canned light tuna, salmon, and shrimp.
		    a. true
		    b. false

d   482   50. Kathy has given birth to a small, low-birthweight infant. Which of the following most likely contributed to this situation?
    a.   smoking
    b.   drug use during pregnancy
    c.   heredity
    d.   poor nutrition

a   484   51. Cindy experienced malnutrition late in her pregnancy. Which of the following organs of the infant will most likely be affected?
    a.   lungs
    b.   heart
    c.   stomach
    d.   brain

d   510   52. Which of the following should be introduced first when feeding a baby?
    a.   pureed vegetables
    b.   citrus fruit juice
    c.   egg white
    d.   rice cereal

c   485   53. A nonpregnant woman requires 1600 calories per day to maintain her desirable body weight. How many calories would she need if she were in the third trimester of pregnancy?
    a.   1900
    b.   1940
    c.   2050
    d.   2125

a   487   54. A nonpregnant woman requires 46 grams of protein per day. How many grams would she need if she became pregnant?
    a.   71
    b.   94
    c.   156
    d.   215

d   489   55. Susie is a pregnant vegetarian who does not consume meat, fish, poultry, or animal products such as dairy foods or eggs. Susie would be at risk for developing a deficiency of:
    a.   vitamin C.
    b.   folate.
    c.   magnesium.
    d.   vitamin B_{12}.

b   509   56. Billy is a 5-month-old infant. Which of the following foods should Billy consume?
    a.   finely chopped meat
    b.   pureed vegetables
    c.   whole cooked egg
    d.   cheese

c	491	57. Nancy weighs 124 pounds and is at an appropriate weight for her height. How much should Nancy weigh at the end of her pregnancy? a. 134 - 139 pounds b. 140 - 149 pounds c. 149 - 159 pounds d. 152 - 164 pounds

d   494

58. You are counseling a pregnant woman who is experiencing "morning sickness." To alleviate this condition you tell her to:
    a.   sip a carbonated beverage before getting out of bed.
    b.   nibble on a soda cracker before getting out of bed.
    c.   try drinking beverages between meals only.
    d.   a and b
    e.   b and c

a   500

59. Beverly consumed 1500 calories daily before she became pregnant. Approximately how many calories should she consume during lactation?
    a.   1830
    b.   1950
    c.   2125
    d.   2250

Controversy Thirteen: Childhood Obesity and Early Chronic Diseases

b   515

60. An estimated 85% of children with type 2 diabetes are:
    a.   physically inactive.
    b.   obese.
    c.   hypertensive.
    d.   Asian.

d   514

61. Which of the following predicts excessive weight gain during childhood and more than doubles the chance that a young child will become an obese adult?
    a.   race and ethnicity
    b.   dietary intake
    c.   physical inactivity
    d.   parental obesity

d   517

62. Which of the following is (are) appropriate for children who are found to have high blood lipids?
    a.   reduction in saturated fat and *trans* fat
    b.   25-35% energy from fat
    c.   reduction in sodium
    d.   a and b
    e.   b and c

a   515

63. Children with the highest carbohydrate intakes, with the exception of added sugars, are leaner than other children.
    a.   true
    b.   false

b   516   64. An adolescent has a total cholesterol level of 180 mg/dl and an LDL of 115 mg/dl. This individual's disease risk would be classified as:
a.   acceptable.
b.   borderline.
c.   normal.
d.   high.

Essay Questions

492   65. Discuss the benefits of physical activity for a pregnant woman.

483-484   66. Why is the mother's nutrition status of importance during the time the placenta is developing?

507   67. Why do many pediatricians advise continued use of infant formula and not cow's milk throughout the first year of life?

494-499   68. Discuss practices which should be avoided during pregnancy, including the rationale.

503   69. Why is the risk of dehydration higher for infants than for adults?

490-491   70. Describe the purpose and components of the Special Supplemental Food Program for Women, Infants, and Children.

497-498   71. Describe alcohol's harmful effects on a fetus.

515-516   72. What are the characteristics of children most likely to develop type 2 diabetes?

515   73. Describe the research findings on the relationship between breastfeeding and degree of body fatness later in life.

Chapter 14 - Child, Teen, and Older Adult

<u>Ans</u>	<u>Page</u>	**<u>Comprehension Level Items</u>**

b 521   1. A child's appetite fluctuates after the age of:
            a.   nine months.
            b.   one year.
            c.   two years.
            d.   three years.

d 522   2. A six-year-old child needs approximately _____ calories a day.
            a.   850
            b.   1000
            c.   1300
            d.   1600

c 532   3. School lunches are designed to provide at least _____ of the recommended intake for each of the nutrients.
            a.   one-fourth
            b.   one-half
            c.   one-third
            d.   two-thirds

a 524   4. Children naturally like nutritious foods in all the food groups with the exception of vegetables.
            a.   true
            b.   false

b 524   5. Which of the following describes foods preferred by children?
            a.   hot vegetables
            b.   mild flavors
            c.   overcooked vegetables
            d.   foods with lumps in them

a 530   6. Television has adverse effects on children's nutrition.
            a.   true
            b.   false

d 530   7. All of the following effects of watching television contribute to obesity **except:**
            a.   it requires no energy and seems to reduce the metabolic rate.
            b.   it consumes time that could be spent in more vigorous activities.
            c.   it correlates with between-meal snacking.
            d.   it presents positive images of overweight people.

e 531   8. To promote dental health, children should be taught to:
            a.   limit between-meal snacking.
            b.   snack on dried fruits.
            c.   eat foods that are swallowed quickly.
            d.   a and b
            e.   a and c

a   528   9. Which of the following is always a component of allergies?
                 a.   antibodies
                 b.   antigens
                 c.   histamine
                 d.   symptoms

c   528   10. The life-threatening food allergy reaction of anaphylactic shock is most often caused by:
                 a.   almonds, yeast breads, and eggs.
                 b.   tomatoes, yeast breads, and peanuts.
                 c.   eggs, peanuts, and milk.
                 d.   soy, fish, and wheat.

b   529   11. Hyperactivity occurs in _____ percent of young, school-age children.
                 a.   1 to 3
                 b.   3 to 5
                 c.   6 to 10
                 d.   7 to 12

d   529-530   12. Which of the following is **not** a cause of "hyper" behavior in children?
                 a.   lack of exercise
                 b.   overstimulation
                 c.   too much television
                 d.   too much sugar

d   529   13. Which of the following is often overlooked as a source of "hyper" behavior in children?
                 a.   food colors
                 b.   additives
                 c.   sugar
                 d.   caffeine

e   535   14. In boys, the adolescent growth spurt peaks at:
                 a.   10.
                 b.   11.
                 c.   12.
                 d.   13.
                 e.   14.

d   535   15. The best way to determine if a teenager is growing normally is to:
                 a.   use growth charts developed for teenagers.
                 b.   calculate the appropriate height and weight based on age.
                 c.   compare him or her with peers.
                 d.   compare his or her height and weight with previous measures taken earlier.

d   535   16. Hormones that regulate the menstrual cycle also alter:
                 a.   glucose tolerance.
                 b.   food intake.
                 c.   iron absorption.
                 d.   a and b
                 e.   b and c

a 536

17. On the average, about _____ of a teenager's total daily energy intake comes from snacks.
    a. one-fourth
    b. one-third
    c. one-eighth
    d. one-half

d 537

18. The woman with PMS should:
    a. try a caffeine-free lifestyle for a while.
    b. get adequate sleep and physical activity.
    c. take megadoses of certain nutrient supplements.
    d. a and b
    e. b and c

b 536

19. Which of the following worsens acne?
    a. greasy foods
    b. stress
    c. cola beverages
    d. nuts

e 525

20. Ways to prevent a child from choking include:
    a. give the child round foods, like grapes and nuts.
    b. avoid dangerous foods such as chips and popcorn.
    c. encourage the child to sit when eating.
    d. a and b
    e. b and c

e 524

21. Which of the following statements is(are) true?
    a. Children should eat at little tables.
    b. Children should be served large portions of foods.
    c. Children should be encouraged to stop eating when they are full.
    d. a and b
    e. a and c

d 544

22. Which of the following have been identified as affecting physiological age?
    a. moderation in alcohol use
    b. regularity of meals
    c. psychological outlook
    d. a and b
    e. b and c

b 539

23. Older adults are not able to gain muscle bulk and strength.
    a. true
    b. false

c 538

24. The fastest growing age group in our society is people:
    a. under 5.
    b. over 55.
    c. over 85.
    d. over 100.

b   538   25. The life expectancy at birth for white women is:
- a.   72 years.
- b.   80 years.
- c.   95 years.
- d.   115 years.

a   539   26. After the age of 50, the intake recommendation for energy assumes a _____ percent reduction in energy output per decade.
- a.   5
- b.   12
- c.   15
- d.   20

b   541   27. Which of the following may speed the progression of osteoarthritis?
- a.   high intake of vitamin E
- b.   low intake of vitamin D
- c.   high intake of vitamin C
- d.   a and b
- e.   a and c

d   541   28. Older adults should:
- a.   consume 14 grams of fiber per 1,000 calories consumed.
- b.   limit the amount of saturated fat in their diets.
- c.   consume more protein than younger adults.
- d.   a and b
- e.   b and c

a   542   29. Absorption of this nutrient appears to increase with aging:
- a.   vitamin A.
- b.   vitamin D.
- c.   calcium.
- d.   iron.

c   543   30. Older adults should drink at least _____ cups of fluid a day to provide needed water.
- a.   3
- b.   5
- c.   6
- d.   8

d   522   31. To determine the fiber needs of a child you would add _____ to the child's age.
- a.   2
- b.   3
- c.   4
- d.   5

d   531   32. An initial goal for obese children is to:
- a.   hold weight steady while they grow taller.
- b.   slow their rate of gain.
- c.   lose weight quickly.
- d.   a and b
- e.   b and c

e   532   33. Authorities recommend limiting fruit juice in children's diets for fear that
                        overconsumption may promote:
                        a.   obesity.
                        b.   hyperactivity.
                        c.   dental caries.
                        d.   a and b
                        e.   a and c

c   539   34. For people over 70, the best health and lowest risk of death have been observed in those
                        who maintain a BMI between:
                        a.   12 and 17.
                        b.   18 and 24.
                        c.   25 and 32.
                        d.   33 and 42.

a   547   35. What is the most important nutrition concern for the person with Alzheimer's disease?
                        a.   prevention of weight loss
                        b.   elimination of dietary aluminum
                        c.   supplementation with zinc
                        d.   treatment with the medicinal herb ginkgo biloba

e.   523   36. Children's intakes of the following nutrient(s) typically fall below recommendations:
                        a.   calcium.
                        b.   vitamin A.
                        c.   zinc.
                        d.   a and b
                        e.   a and c

a   522   37. To prevent iron deficiency, children's foods must deliver from 7 to 10 milligrams of iron
                        per day.
                        a.   true
                        b.   false

a   531   38. Nutrients missed from a skipped breakfast won't be made up at lunch and dinner but will
                        be left out completely that day.
                        a.   true
                        b.   false

d   542   39. To prevent early onset of cataracts the diet should provide an ample supply of:
                        a.   vitamin C.
                        b.   vitamin E.
                        c.   vitamin A.
                        d.   a or b
                        e.   b or c

a   528   40. By 2006, food labels must announce the presence of common allergens in plain
                        language, using the names of the eight most common allergy-causing foods.
                        a.   true
                        b.   false

Application Level Items

a   525

41. Which of the following would be the most appropriate snack for an active, normal weight child?
    a. ice cream
    b. candy
    c. Oreo cookies
    d. cola

b   524

42. Which of the following foods would be most acceptable to a child?
    a. hot vegetable soup
    b. lightly crunchy steamed carrots
    c. mashed potatoes with lumps
    d. hot broccoli with cheese sauce

e   525

43. Which of the following children is(are) most at risk for choking?
    a. Susie, who is sitting down and eating tender beef strips
    b. Charles, who is snacking on popcorn while watching television
    c. Billy, who is eating while running around the table
    d. a and b
    e. b and c

b   526-527

44. A parent who wishes to protect her child from lead toxicity would do all of the following **except:**
    a. prevent the child from chewing on old painted surfaces.
    b. feed the child additional protein.
    c. wash the child's hands, bottles and toys often.
    d. make sure the child gets an adequate calcium intake.

a   528

45. Tommy consumed a breakfast consisting of eggs, whole-grain toast with cheese, and orange juice. Shortly thereafter, Tommy experienced an allergic reaction. This reaction was most likely caused by:
    a. eggs
    b. whole-grain toast
    c. cheese
    d. orange juice

d   529-530

46. Normal, everyday causes of "hyper" behavior in children include all of the following **except:**
    a. desire for attention.
    b. lack of sleep.
    c. overstimulation.
    d. too much exercise.

c   531

47. Which of the following foods should be used infrequently in order to control dental caries?
    a. carrot sticks
    b. bagels
    c. chocolate milk
    d. plain yogurt

d   536-537   48. A teenager consumes a fast food meal consisting of a hamburger, chocolate shake, and french fries. In order to consume an adequate diet, which of the following should be chosen at other meals during the day?

      a.   foods high in vitamins A and C
      b.   good fiber sources
      c.   foods high in energy
      d.   a and b
      e.   b and c

b   535   49. Joe is a 15 year-old active male. However, his parents are concerned that Joe is not growing properly. To assess his growth, Joe's parents should:

      a.   compare Joe's height and weight to his best friends'.
      b.   compare his height and weight with previous measures taken at intervals.
      c.   compare Joe's height and weight to those on growth charts.
      d.   a and b
      e.   b and c

c   541, 543   50. Lois is a 65-year-old female who participates in an exercise class at least three times a week. In addition, she drinks six glasses of water each day and consumes a lot of fresh fruits and vegetables and whole-grain breads and cereals. Lois has high blood pressure, takes medication for her hypertension, and experiences constipation frequently. Which of the following is the most likely cause of her constipation?

      a.   low fiber intake
      b.   inadequate exercise
      c.   medications
      d.   low fluid intake

Controversy Fourteen: Nutrient-Drug Interactions: Who Should Be Concerned?

c   553   51. Which of the following can increase the anti-blood clotting effect of aspirin?

      a.   nicotine
      b.   antibiotics
      c.   ginkgo biloba
      d.   antacids

a   552   52. People taking two or more drugs at the same time are more vulnerable to nutrient-drug interactions.

      a.   true
      b.   false

e   553   53. Which of the following can interfere with the absorption of certain antibiotics?

      a.   dairy products
      b.   nicotine gum
      c.   calcium-fortified juices
      d.   a and b
      e.   a and c

b   554   54. People who take aspirin regularly should eat _____ foods regularly.

      a.   fiber-rich
      b.   iron-rich
      c.   vitamin C-rich
      d.   calcium-rich

b   552   55. Medical drugs do only good, but do not harm.
         a.   true
         b.   false

Essay Questions

530-531   56. Discuss the impact of television on children's eating behaviors and nutrition status.

531   57. Describe characteristics of children who do not eat breakfast compared to those of their well-fed peers.

542   58. Why do older adults face a greater risk of vitamin D deficiency than younger people?

542   59. Describe the theory that links dietary composition with macular degeneration.

538-540   60. Why do energy needs often decrease with advancing age?

543   61. Why is dehydration a major risk for older adults?

543   62. Describe factors that make iron deficiency likely in older people.

553-554   63. Describe how chronic laxative use can lead to malnutrition.

557   64. Describe how the nutrient intakes of smokers and non-smokers differ.

533   65. How does the dietary composition of adolescents who eat their evening meals at home with their families differ from that of adolescents who do not?

Chapter 15 - Hunger and the
Global Environment

Ans.	Page	Comprehension Level Items

c   562

1. Which of the following trends is currently taking place and projected for the next decade?
   - a. Food producing land is increasing.
   - b. Fuel use is decreasing.
   - c. Supplies of fresh water are dwindling.
   - d. Air quality is improving.

b   574

2. The U.S. government's Energy Star logo is from the:
   - a. Food and Consumer Service.
   - b. Environmental Protection Agency.
   - c. Food and Drug Administration.
   - d. World Health Organization.

a   571

3. When people obtain better access to health care, education, and family planning, the death rate falls.
   - a. true
   - b. false

d   563

4. Chronic hunger causes many deaths worldwide, especially among:
   - a. older adults.
   - b. women.
   - c. newborns.
   - d. children.

a   574

5. Energy Star products range from large appliances to light bulbs and building materials.
   - a. true
   - b. false

d   563

6. Which of the following segments are included in the chronic poor category?
   - a. the homeless
   - b. migrant workers
   - c. displaced farm families
   - d. a and b
   - e. b and c

b   574

7. All of the following results in the permanent loss of rainforests **except:**
   - a. corned beef.
   - b. cashews.
   - c. pet foods.
   - d. canned stews.

b   574

8. If you are a meat eater, which of the following recommendations would you follow to be environmentally conscious?
   - a. Eat beef less often than pork.
   - b. Select chicken from local farms.
   - c. Choose canned stew beef.
   - d. a and b
   - e. a and c

a   569   9. Which of the following species of fish is **not** endangered by overfishing?
   a.   bass
   b.   shark
   c.   swordfish
   d.   tuna

c   574   10. Which of the following would you choose in order to save costs in fuel and protect the environment?
   a.   frozen fish
   b.   fish flown in from far away
   c.   small fish
   d.   refrigerated fish

d   574   11. Switching to local foods grown close to home results in:
   a.   money savings.
   b.   nutritional advantages.
   c.   healthier products.
   d.   environmental advantages.

c   574   12. Which of the following food packages is best for the environment?
   a.   foam trays
   b.   glass jars
   c.   reusable ones
   d.   plastic bottles

b   574   13. Which of the following packaging techniques for processed foods is the most environmentally advantageous?
   a.   juices in small individual cartons
   b.   eggs in pressed fiber cartons
   c.   grain products in separate little packages
   d.   meats in foam trays

c   574   14. Which of the following is the best choice for grocery bags?
   a.   recyclable plastic bags
   b.   paper bags
   c.   reusable shopping bags
   d.   non-recyclable plastic bags

a   574   15. Which of the following cooking methods wastes the most fuel?
   a.   baking
   b.   pressure cooking
   c.   stir-frying
   d.   microwaving

d   574   16. Which of the following cooking aids is the most environmentally benign?
   a.   plastic storage bags
   b.   sponges
   c.   paper towels
   d.   cloth towels

b   575   17. Which of the following is one of the most substantial consumers of energy in most people's homes?
- a.   electric can openers
- b.   refrigerators
- c.   electric mixers
- d.   microwave ovens

e   575   18. To minimize the energy a refrigerator uses, you would:
- a.   set the refrigerator at 25 to 28º F.
- b.   clean the coils regularly.
- c.   set the freezer at 0º F.
- d.   a and b
- e.   b and c

c   575   19. To save energy, you would set the water heater at:
- a.   100 - 110º F.
- b.   110 - 120º F.
- c.   120 - 130º F.
- d.   130 - 140º F.

a   568   20. At the present rate of growth, the world's population will soon outstrip the current rate of food production.
- a.   true
- b.   false

b   567   21. Natural causes of famine have become more important in recent years than the social causes.
- a.   true
- b.   false

d   567   22. Over _____ million people, mostly women and children, suffer from malnutrition.
- a.   100
- b.   200
- c.   500
- d.   800

e   563   23. The predominant form of hunger in the United States today is:
- a.   intermittent.
- b.   caused by lack of food nearby to purchase.
- c.   caused by lack of money.
- d.   a and b
- e.   a and c

a   563, 565   24. The primary cause of hunger is:
- a.   poverty.
- b.   mental illness.
- c.   depression.
- d.   illness.

d   563   25. Examples of the so called working poor in the United States include:
- a.   displaced farm families.
- b.   white collar workers forced out of their professions.
- c.   migrant workers.
- d.   a and b
- e.   b and c

d   564   26. Food stamp recipients may use their coupons like cash to purchase:
- a. vegetables.
- b. seeds.
- c. cleaning items.
- d. a and b
- e. b and c

a   564-565   27. Federal programs to relieve hunger are not fully successful in preventing hunger.
- a. true
- b. false

a   564   28. Participation in the WIC Program during pregnancy is associated with increased weight and longer gestation.
- a. true
- b. false

a   563   29. Hunger is not always easy to recognize.
- a. true
- b. false

c   570   30. Which of the following represents the only way to enable the world's food output to keep pace with people's growing numbers?
- a. increased water supplies
- b. decreased air pollution
- c. population stabilization
- d. additional farm land

b   574   31. The largest source of air pollution in the U.S. is:
- a. airplanes.
- b. motor vehicles.
- c. factories.
- d. trains.

a   562-563   32. The single greatest cause of preventable brain damage and mental retardation is:
- a. iodine deficiency.
- b. vitamin A deficiency.
- c. iron deficiency.
- d. folate deficiency.

d   564   33. One out of every _____ Americans receives food assistance of some kind.
- a. three
- b. four
- c. five
- d. six

c   567   34. Which of the following groups is the first to suffer when crops fail or war and violence erupt in an already impoverished area?
- a. children
- b. the elderly
- c. women
- d. infants

e   572   35. To solve the world's environmental, poverty, and hunger problems, rich nations must:
                  a.   stem their wasteful and polluting use of the resources.
                  b.   gain control of their population growth.
                  c.   stem the use of energy.
                  d.   a and b
                  e.   a and c

c   564   36. Which of the following programs is the centerpiece of U.S. food programs for low-income families?
                  a.   WIC Program
                  b.   Community Supplemental Food Program
                  c.   Food Stamp Program
                  d.   Senior Nutrition Program

d   569-570 37. To protect yourself from consuming too much _____, you would limit your consumption of swordfish, king mackerel and shark.
                  a.   lead
                  b.   arsenic
                  c.   iodine
                  d.   mercury

a   561   38. Living in a country at war or lack of transportation can lead to:
                  a.   food poverty.
                  b.   food shortage.
                  c.   food insecurity.
                  d.   food recovery.

b   564   39. Facilities that collect and distribute food donations to authorized organizations feeding the hungry are called:
                  a.   food recovery centers.
                  b.   food banks.
                  c.   food pantries.
                  d.   emergency kitchens.

a   561   40. The concentration of carbon dioxide in the atmosphere is now 26% higher than 200 years ago.
                  a.   true
                  b.   false

Application Level Items

c   574   41. In order to be an environmentally conscious shopper you would:
                  a.   drive to the grocery store three times per week.
                  b.   stock up on canned beef products like chili.
                  c.   consume more plant foods than animal products.
                  d.   eat large fish versus smaller ones.

b   574   42. You decide to choose more local food products rather than choosing those shipped from long distances. By doing this you are:
                  a.   saving money.
                  b.   helping the environment.
                  c.   creating more jobs in your local community.
                  d.   contributing to world hunger.

c   574   43. Which of the following represents environmentally sound food packaging?
        a.   labels which boast of environmentally sound packaging
        b.   ears of corn packaged in individual packages
        c.   bulk items with minimal packaging
        d.   milk in individual cartons

d   574   44. By not choosing overly packaged items you are:
        a.   contributing to the destruction of fisheries.
        b.   contributing to the death of wildlife.
        c.   alleviating one possible cause of cancer.
        d.   helping to save the environment from pollution.

d   574   45. Which of the following represents the most energy-efficient way of cooking vegetables?
        a.   stir-frying
        b.   microwaving
        c.   oven roasting
        d.   a and b
        e.   b and c

b   574   46. The best method to keep food from sticking that is also the most advantageous from an environmental perspective is to:
        a.   use a canned cooking spray.
        b.   apply a little oil by hand.
        c.   use aluminum foil.
        d.   apply shortening using a paper towel.

b   574   47. Which of the following food preparation methods would you use to save energy?
        a.   beat eggs with an electric mixer
        b.   cut vegetables using a sharp knife
        c.   chop meats using a food processor
        d.   mix up a milkshake using an electric blender

d   570-571   48. Which of the following results in the slowest rate of population growth?
        a.   economic growth and improvement in living standards
        b.   have all groups share resources relatively equally
        c.   have resources unevenly distributed
        d.   a and b
        e.   b and c

e   572   49. To solve the world's environmental, poverty, and hunger problems, poor nations must:
        a.   gain control of their population growth.
        b.   slow and reverse the destruction of their environmental resources.
        c.   stem their wasteful and polluting use of resources and energy.
        d.   a and c
        e.   a and b

Controversy Fifteen: Agribusiness and Food Production: How to Go Forward?

d   582-583   50. To eat lower on the food chain you would:
        a.   choose more grains.
        b.   consume more vegetables.
        c.   eat more beef.
        d.   a and b
        e.   b and c

d   578   51. Long-term effects of irrigation include:
                    a.   the soil becomes more salty.
                    b.   the water supply becomes depleted.
                    c.   the plant growth is facilitated.
                    d.   a and b
                    e.   b and c

a   579   52. More land in the United States is used to produce feed grains for livestock than is used to produce grain for people.
                    a.   true
                    b.   false

b   579   53. In the United States, the food industry's energy consumption is about _____ percent of all the energy the nation uses.
                    a.   10
                    b.   20
                    c.   30
                    d.   40

e   580-581 54. Alternative, sustainable agricultural practices include:
                    a.   rotating crops.
                    b.   using fertilizers generously.
                    c.   feeding livestock on the open range.
                    d.   a and b
                    e.   a and c

c   582   55. Which of the following foods requires the least energy to produce?
                    a.   fruits
                    b.   vegetables
                    c.   grains
                    d.   animal protein

Essay Questions

561, 563   56. Describe what is meant by food poverty, including its major cause.

564-565   57. What is food recovery and how does it help communities reduce hunger and improve nutrition?

571-573   58. Identify and describe the solutions to solving the world's environmental, poverty and hunger problems.

570-571   59. Explain how poverty leads to overpopulation.

569-571   60. Describe what is meant by the statement that *"poverty causes environmental ruin, and the ruin leads to hunger"*?

564-565   61. Describe some of the U.S. food programs directed at stopping domestic hunger.

572, 581   62. Explain what is meant by the term *"sustainable."*

580-581   63. Compare and contrast high-input and low-input agricultural techniques.

580-581   64. What is meant by the term *"precision agriculture"*?

567-568   65. Why are women in developing countries being targeted as direct recipients of food relief?

Lesson 1: Nutrition Basics

Ans	Objective	
b	13/V1	1. The study of how a person's genes interact with nutrients is termed a. genetic counseling. b. nutritional genomics. c. genetic metabolomics. d. nutritional nucleic acid pool.
c	2/V2	2. The nutrient that provides us with fuel for the brain and nervous system is a. protein. b. fat. c. carbohydrate. d. vitamins.
b	2/V2	3. Proteins are considered the a. main source of quick energy for the body. b. building blocks of life. c. activator of chemical reactions in the body. d. best source of concentrated energy.
c	2/V2	4. The nutrient that provides the most concentrated form of energy and carries essential vitamins along with it is a. carbohydrate. b. minerals. c. fat. d. protein.
a	2/V2	5. Nearly every chemical reaction in the body occurs in an environment consisting of a. water. b. minerals. c. carbohydrate. d. fat.
b	13/V3	6. What foods are found at the base of the Food Guide Pyramid? a. Fruits and vegetables b. Grains and cereals c. Dairy products d. Meat products
d	13/V3	7. The top of the Pyramid consists of a. foods that supply many kcalories but few nutrients. b. high fat and high sugar foods. c. "junk" foods. d. all of the above.
d	13/V3	8. Vegetarians can apply the Food Guide Pyramid by substituting a. legumes for protein. b. seeds/nuts for protein. c. peanut butter for protein. d. all of the above.

c   9/V3   9.   A serving of meat is
                              a.   what you typically get at a restaurant.
                              b.   what most people typically eat.
                              c.   3-4 ounces.
                              d.   6-8 ounces.

b   6/V4   10. All of the following are health concerns of each Pathway subject who will be
                              followed for one year EXCEPT
                              a.   weight control.
                              b.   cancer.
                              c.   diabetes.
                              d.   high blood cholesterol.

Objective	**Q#**	
13/V1	11.	What was developed by nutrition scientists in 1940 to help the nation prevent deficiencies?
13/V3	12.	According to the Food Guide Pyramid, what constitutes a serving of milk?
13/V3	13.	According to the Food Guide Pyramid, what constitutes a serving of fruit?
6/V4	14.	What are the three health concerns of the Pathway subjects being profiled for one year?

Answer

11.   Recommended Dietary Allowances (RDA)

12.   Milk = 1 cup

13.   1/2 cup sliced (or one medium whole fruit, such as an apple or banana)

14.   Type II diabetes (diabetes), high blood cholesterol (CVD, heart disease), and weight loss (weight control)

Lesson 2: The Digestive System

Ans	Objective	
c	7/V1	1. What is the very first thing you should do if you suspect someone is choking on food? a. Perform the Heimlich maneuver. b. Strike the person sharply on the back. c. Ask the person to try to talk. d. Attempt to dislodge the food with your fingers.
b	7/V1	2. The life-saving technique that utilizes an upper abdominal thrust to try to dislodge food from the airway of someone who is choking is known as a. CPR. b. Heimlich maneuver. c. Mouth-to-mouth resuscitation. d. All of the above.
c	7/V2	3. Which of the following foods that delay gastric emptying may cause an increase in belching? a. Carbohydrate b. Protein c. Fat d. Calcium
b	7/V3	4. The use of an antacid is indicated primarily for which of the following conditions? a. Excessive gas b. Acid indigestion c. Excessive belching d. Bloating
c	7/V3	5. An effective way of treating heartburn or acid indigestion is to a. drink milk. b. hold your breath. c. take antacids. d. drink water.
c	7/V4	6. Which of the following is most likely to result from insufficient intake of fiber? a. Diarrhea b. Bloating c. Constipation d. Pancreatitis
a	7/V4	7. People are said to be constipated when they experience a. painful or difficult bowel movements. b. more than a day or two without a bowel movement. c. soft or watery bowel movements with little notice. d. none of the above.

b   7/V5   8. Peptic ulcers can be caused by
  a. acidic foods.
  b. bacteria.
  c. spicy foods.
  d. smoking.

Objective	Q#	
7/V1	9.	The most obvious sign of choking is that the person cannot
7/V2	10.	The function of belching is to rid the small intestine or stomach of
7/V2	11.	Flatus (gas from the lower abdomen) is produced by fermentation of undigested food products caused by
7/V3	12.	The greatest danger from vomiting is
7/V3	13.	The relaxation of the gastroesophageal sphincter which produces a burning sensation in the esophagus is called

Answer

09. speak (make a sound, cough).

10. carbon dioxide (gas).

11. bacteria (GI tract or colon).

12. dehydration.

13. acid indigestion (heartburn).

Lesson 3: Carbohydrates: Simple and Complex

Ans	Objective		
c	1/V1	1.	Athletes or active individuals who require large amounts of energy should consume a diet high in a. protein. b. fat. c. carbohydrate. d. water.
c	1/V1	2.	Tennis players require immediate bursts of energy which come from a. amino acids. b. fatty acids. c. glycogen. d. glycerol.
b	8/V2	3.	The hormone that is secreted when blood glucose is high is a. glucagon. b. insulin. c. thyroxin. d. epinephrine.
a	9/V3	4.	Which of the following statements is the most accurate regarding studies documenting hyperactivity and sugar intake in children? a. There is very little evidence to support the statement that sugar causes hyperactivity. b. There is considerable evidence that sugar and hyperactivity are positively linked. c. There is substantial scientific proof that sugar causes hyperactivity. d. None of the above.
d	9/V3	5.	Parents should limit a child's intake of sugar because a. it causes hyperactivity. b. it takes the place of healthier foods. c. it may adversely affect the child's growth. d. b and c.

Objective	Q#	
1/V1	6.	High carbohydrate diets have been shown to increase an athlete's
8/V2	7.	Hypoglycemia refers to a low level of

Answer

6. endurance. (stamina, energy, aerobic capacity)

7. blood glucose (blood sugar).

Lesson 4: Carbohydrates: Fiber

<u>Ans</u>	<u>Objective</u>	

d	8/V1	1. When whole wheat is refined, the part(s) of the grain that is(are) removed is(are) the
		  a. bran.
		  b. germ.
		  c. endosperm.
		  d. a and b.

c	8/V1	2. When we eat refined white bread, the part of the wheat grain that we are eating is the
		  a. bran.
		  b. germ.
		  c. endosperm.
		  d. all of the above.

c	4/V2	3. Which of the following conditions/diseases does fiber NOT protect against?
		  a. Obesity
		  b. Cancer
		  c. Cataracts
		  d. Hypertension

c	4/V2	4. When people go on a high-fiber diet, by what percent can they lower blood cholesterol?
		  a. 5-10%
		  b. 15-20%
		  c. 20-30%
		  d. More than 50%

d	4/V2	5. High-fiber foods are helpful for people who wish to lose weight because they
		  a. take longer to eat.
		  b. are more filling.
		  c. provide few calories.
		  d. all of the above.

d	4/V3	6. High levels of dietary fiber intake may protect us against
		  a. colon cancer.
		  b. rectal cancer.
		  c. breast cancer.
		  d. all of the above.

d	4/V4	7. People with inflammatory bowel diseases could possibly benefit from higher fiber diets because fiber
		  a. can preserve the mucosa of the colon.
		  b. can improve peristaltic action of the GI tract.
		  c. will cause more frequent and regular bowel movements.
		  d. a and b.

a	4/V4	8. In patients with inflammatory bowel disease or Crohn's disease, high-fiber intakes may benefit them by
		  a. normalizing the intestinal contents throughout the colon.
		  b. causing them to have lower blood pressure which accompanies Crohn's disease.
		  c. preventing weight gain that accompanies inflammatory bowel disease.
		  d. all of the above.

b	5/V6	9.	The newest dietary recommendation regarding fiber for people with type II diabetes is that fiber intake

9. The newest dietary recommendation regarding fiber for people with type II diabetes is that fiber intake
   a. should be lower than for the general population to prevent constipation.
   b. should be increased by eating more whole fruits, whole grains, and legumes.
   c. is not necessary to address, whereas sugar intake is important to address.
   d. none of the above.

a   5/V6   10. In order to increase fiber intake, people with type II diabetes would be encouraged to eat all of the following foods EXCEPT
   a. orange juice.
   b. whole oranges.
   c. potatoes.
   d. broccoli.

Objective	**Q#**	
8/V1	11.	How much fiber per serving is found in whole wheat kernels and in refined wheat flour, respectively?
4/V2	12.	List three of the "famous five" conditions that fiber is known to protect against.
4/V2	13.	When people go on high-fiber diets and reduce their blood cholesterol by as little as 10%, they can reduce their risk for heart attack by
4/V3	14.	Against what type of cancer might high intakes of dietary fiber offer protection?
5/V5	15.	When people increase their dietary fiber intake, they must also increase their intake of
5/V5	16.	Cite one symptom associated with overdosing on dietary fiber.

Answer

11.   9 grams and 1 gram

12.   Answers must include three of the following:
*Heart disease   *Cancer
*Obesity   *Diabetes
*High blood pressure

13.   20%.

14.   Answer may include any of the following:
* Colon   * Rectal
* Breast

15.   water (fluids).

16.   Answer may be any of the following:
* Abdominal bloating   * Gas
* Diarrhea ("runs")   * Constipation

Lesson 5: Fats: The Lipid Family

Ans	**Objective**		

b   8/V1

1. The best energy source for strenuous, aerobic type activities, such as hiking, is
   a. phospholipids.
   b. triglycerides.
   c. carbohydrates.
   d. sterols.

d   8/V1

2. Foods that are good choices for an activity such as hiking include
   a. high fat foods.
   b. peanut butter.
   c. salami.
   d. all of the above.

d   8/V1

3. Foods such as peanuts, GORP, cheese, and salami are good choices for hiking because they
   a. provide concentrated energy.
   b. are easily packed.
   c. are high-fat foods.
   d. all of the above.

d   8/V2

4. Lipoproteins
   a. transport lipids through a watery medium, the blood.
   b. are protein-based vehicles for the transport of lipids.
   c. are composed of lipids and proteins.
   d. all of the above.

a   8/V2

5. Lipids need a transport carrier
   a. to move them through the bloodstream.
   b. in case they are not absorbed in the stomach.
   c. because lipids are water soluble.
   d. none of the above.

d   10/V3

6. Blood cholesterol is impacted by
   a. lifestyle.
   b. nutrition.
   c. heredity.
   d. all of the above.

b   10/V3

7. Cholesterol is necessary for the production of many other compounds in the body but can become harmful when blood levels
   a. exceed 135 mg/dl.
   b. exceed the body's ability to use it.
   c. can only be controlled through medications.
   d. a and b.

d   10/V3

8. What changes in lifestyle could bring about reductions in blood cholesterol?
   a. Regular aerobic-type exercise
   b. Restricting total fat
   c. Restricting saturated fat
   d. All of the above

a   11/V4   9. Fat substitutes were developed to
- a. help control kcalories in foods.
- b. help people reduce body fat.
- c. make foods taste better.
- d. all of the above.

b   12/V4   10. A fat substitute that has recently been approved by the FDA is
- a. Simplesse.
- b. Olestra.
- c. Fatestra.
- d. Simpola.

a   11/V4   11. Simplesse is a fat substitute made of
- a. protein particles.
- b. whipped egg whites.
- c. blended sugars.
- d. sugar with a fatty acid.

d   11/V5   12. Blood triglyceride levels can be reduced by reducing which of the following foods?
- a. Alcohol
- b. Sweets
- c. Complex carbohydrates
- d. a and b

a   11/V5   13. The recommendation for blood cholesterol is
- a. less than 200 mg/dl.
- b. 210-150 mg/dl.
- c. under 100 mg/dl.
- d. 250-285 mg/dl.

d   11/V5   14. Someone with high blood cholesterol would be advised to frequently monitor and reduce
- a. dietary cholesterol intake.
- b. total fat intake.
- c. saturated fat intake.
- d. all of the above.

Lesson 6 : Fats: Health Effects

<u>Ans</u>	<u>Objective</u>	
c	3/V1	1. The American Heart Association recommends the percentage of total calories that come from fat should not exceed a. 10%. b. 20%. c. 30%. d. 40%.
b	3/V1	2. From an optimum health perspective, the best type of fat is a. polyunsaturated fat. b. monounsaturated fat. c. saturated fat. d. none of the above.
b	3/V1	3. What is the recommended intake for saturated fat? a. 10% or more b. No more than 10% c. 12% - 14% d. Less than 30%
d	8/V2	4. A person can reduce fat in a diet that has beef as its base by a. selecting leaner cuts of meat. b. choosing chicken or fish occasionally. c. becoming a vegan-vegetarian. d. a and b.
a	8/V2	5. Meat-eaters can reduce fat in their diets by a. baking, broiling, or braising meats. b. frying or sauteing meats in olive oil. c. using regular hamburger for meat loaf. d. selecting regular hamburger instead of sirloin steaks.
d	8/V2	6. Some people who eat high-meat diets may have a greater risk for a. cardiovascular disease. b. colon cancer. c. obesity. d. all of the above.
d	8/V2	7. If a person is performing physical labor at a very high level of intensity and/or for very long periods of time, the person could a. increase total kcalories. b. consume more fat than the average person. c. expend more calories than the average person. d. all of the above.
d	8/V3	8. The foundation of a Mediterranean diet consists of a. olive oil as the primary fat. b. fruits and vegetables as the base. c. lots of grains and breads. d. all of the above.

b	8/V3	9.	Most people who consume a Mediterranean diet typically

b 8/V3 9. Most people who consume a Mediterranean diet typically
   a. suffer from obesity.
   b. do not suffer from cardiovascular disease.
   c. show signs of type II diabetes.
   d. do not develop lung cancer.

c 8/V3 10. Problems such as cardiovascular disease, diabetes, obesity, and some cancers seem to occur less often in populations who consume a typical
   a. American diet.
   b. American Indian diet.
   c. Mediterranean diet.
   d. none of the above.

a 8/V3 11. Olive oil and seafood have been shown to
   a. decrease risk for cardiovascular disease.
   b. increase risk for obesity.
   c. increase risk for type II diabetes.
   d. decrease risk for skin cancer.

a 9/V4 12. If you wanted to reduce the fat and kcalories in a 10 oz. portion of prime rib, you could
   a. eat 5 oz. and save the rest for the next day.
   b. cut away all visible fat but still eat the 10 oz.
   c. refuse to eat any of the meat.
   d. either a or b.

d 9/V4 13. If you wanted to reduce the fat and kcalories in mashed potatoes prepared with milk and butter, you could
   a. use instant mashed potatoes.
   b. mash the potatoes with water and use butter flavoring instead.
   c. use skim milk and low-fat margarine instead.
   d. b and c.

a 9/V4 14. Over a period of time, if one were to consistently reduce fat in the diet, one could
   a. lose body fat.
   b. gain lean muscle.
   c. increase aerobic capacity.
   d. none of the above.

d 4/V5 15. People who have type II diabetes can reduce fat intake by
   a. eating more fruits and vegetables.
   b. drinking skim milk.
   c. eating smaller portions of meat.
   d. all of the above.

a 4/V5 16. Reducing fat intake for a person with type II diabetes can be accomplished by
   a. increasing fruits and vegetables.
   b. increasing meat portions.
   c. decreasing breads and grains.
   d. a and c.

Lesson 7: Protein: Form and Function

Ans	Objective		

d   6/V1

1. Which of the following statements is accurate regarding protein?
   a. "Protein builds muscle bulk and strength."
   b. "Protein supplements provide an important energy boost."
   c. "People in North America don't suffer from protein deficiencies."
   d. None of the above.

d   6/V1

2. Protein is needed for normal development of cells and muscle mass but excessive amounts of protein
   a. are even better and will bring faster results.
   b. will not significantly increase the building of body tissue.
   c. won't add significant strength to the body.
   d. b and c.

b   6/V1

3. In order to gain muscle size and strength, it is necessary to
   a. increase protein intake well above the RDA.
   b. train intensely with adequate rest periods in between.
   c. train every day at the highest intensity possible.
   d. all of the above.

d   9/V2

4. High intakes of animal protein sources are associated with serious health risks such as
   a. increased cardiovascular disease.
   b. colon cancer.
   c. breast cancer.
   d. all of the above.

c   9/V2

5. Cardiovascular disease, colon cancer, and breast cancer risks have been shown to increase with diets high in
   a. all protein.
   b. plant protein.
   c. animal protein.
   d. all of the above.

d   8/V3

6. Kwashiorkor, a condition frequently found in the Republic of Guinea, is characterized by
   a. a diet lacking in a direct source of protein such as meat.
   b. a starch-based diet.
   c. a diet consisting of water and oil with lots of rice.
   d. all of the above.

d   8/V3

7. Marasmus can be characterized as a condition in which
   a. overeating results in bloating and edema.
   b. the person is starving from total malnutrition.
   c. the immune system is impaired, allowing for microbe attack.
   d. b and c.

d   8/V3

8. In the U.S., protein-energy malnutrition can be seen most often in which of the following populations?
   a. Cancer patients
   b. AIDS patients
   c. Inner city children
   d. All of the above

c   8/V4   9. What percent of protein is provided by the School Lunch Program funded by the federal government?
a. 10%
b. 30%
c. 50%
d. 100%

d   8/V4   10. The primary component(s) of the School Lunch Program that help prevent protein-energy malnutrition in U.S. school children is(are)
a. meat or meat alternates.
b. milk.
c. pasta and breads.
d. a and b.

d   9/V5   11. For someone who has high blood cholesterol, protein foods should
a. come from plant sources rather than animal sources.
b. represent the bulk of the diet.
c. not be a concern if they are eating from the Food Guide Pyramid.
d. a and c.

b   9/V5   12. The best examples of protein sources for people with high blood cholesterol are
a. meat and fish.
b. beans and rice.
c. milk and dairy products.
d. any of the above.

Lesson 8: The Protein Continuum

Ans	Objective		
a	5/V1	1.	Protein intakes may increase as a result of illness as well as

a   5/V1   1. Protein intakes may increase as a result of illness as well as
   a. when women are lactating.
   b. during moderate anaerobic activity.
   c. during times of optimal health.
   d. any of the above.

d   5/V1   2. What is the typical protein intake for adults living in the U.S.?
   a. 100% of the RDA for protein
   b. Between 80-120 grams/day
   c. Two to three times the RDA for protein
   d. b and c

d   7/V2   3. People who consume a diet in which meat is the primary source of protein are
   a. at less risk for cancer than vegetarians.
   b. thought to be at greater risk for cancer than vegetarians.
   c. more likely to develop heart disease than vegetarians.
   d. b and c.

c   7/V2   4. What vitamin does meat provide that is NOT in plant-based diets?
   a. vitamin A.
   b. vitamin D.
   c. vitamin B_{12}.
   d. riboflavin.

d   7/V2   5. Reasons why people choose to become vegetarians include
   a. ethical issues surrounding animal rights.
   b. personal health reasons.
   c. weight loss.
   d. any of the above.

c   7/V2   6. People who are semi-vegetarians eat
   a. meat or animal products every other day.
   b. animal foods most of the time except on religious holidays.
   c. meat, milk, or eggs only periodically.
   d. any of the above.

d   6/V3   7. How can people reduce the amount of animal protein they eat daily?
   a. Eat meat less often and in smaller portions.
   b. Choose meat alternates as protein sources.
   c. Select plant-based protein sources occasionally.
   d. Any of the above.

a   6/V3   8. For people who wish to lose weight, most experts might advise them to
   a. consider eating more vegetarian protein sources.
   b. stay at the top of the Food Guide Pyramid for food choices.
   c. focus on the middle of the Food Guide Pyramid for choices.
   d. eat only plant-based proteins, completely eliminating meat.

Lesson 9: Metabolism

Ans	Objective		
d	1/V1	1.	A power plant and the body's metabolism are similar in that both

        a. generate energy.
        b. store unused energy.
        c. release energy when needed.
        d. all of the above.

c   13/V3   2. If you take in a large number of calories but exercise vigorously and regularly, you will probably
        a. gain weight.
        b. lose weight.
        c. maintain weight.
        d. none of the above.

d   13/V3   3. Every time you put on an extra pound of body fat, you can
        a. increase blood pressure.
        b. decrease blood pressure.
        c. become more susceptible to some cancers.
        d. a and c.

d   11/V4   4. During a prolonged fast, the brain
        a. adapts to using 20-30 mg of glucose per minute.
        b. relies mostly on ketone bodies.
        c. is less reliant on glucose to function.
        d. all of the above.

d   14/V5   5. Chronic alcohol use affects metabolism and the energy pathway by
        a. disrupting liver function.
        b. damaging the liver.
        c. leading to malnutrition.
        d. all of the above.

Objective

10/V2   6. The nutrient that is the most calorie dense on a weight-to-weight basis is

13/V3   7. For a person with diabetes, the metabolic rate can be increased through

11/V4   8. Long-term fasting can cause the heart muscle to

              9. How does alcohol intake impact the body's use of B vitamins?

Q#   Answers

6. fat (fatty acids, triglycerides).

7. exercise (physical activity).

8. diminish in size (atrophy, get smaller, shrink).

9. Prevents absorption (depletes vitamins)

Lesson 10: Weight Control: Energy Regulation

Ans	Objective		

d   3/V1   1.

Factors that affect food intake include
a. genetics.
b. hunger and appetite.
c. age.
d. all of the above.

a   3/V1   2.

When people eat dessert even if they are stuffed from a meal, they are responding to a cue to eat known as
a. sensory specific satiety.
b. gluttony syndrome.
c. over-indulgence syndrome.
d. appestatic satiety.

b   3/V1   3.

Internal cues regarding eating should tell people to
a. eat when they are full, stop when they are satisfied.
b. eat when they are hungry, stop when they are satisfied.
c. continue eating beyond satiety, ignoring feelings.
d. all of the above.

c   11/V2   4.

What population has been the primary target of body image idealization especially in the U.S. culture?
a. Males
b. Adolescents
c. Females
d. Children

a   11/V2   5.

Glamorizing thinness through the media has been historically aimed at what population?
a. Upper middle class white females
b. Lower socioeconomic groups
c. Higher socioeconomic white males
d. Middle class non-Caucasian adolescents

a   11/V2   6.

Even though men are not exempt from the pressure brought on by the media to be thin, it appears that men as opposed to women
a. derive a sense of self-esteem not based on size or shape.
b. realize the difference between media hype and truth.
c. are able to identify better ways to lose weight.
d. all of the above.

c   7/V3   7.

Body weight that is associated with the lowest mortality or minimum death is referred to by experts as
a. ideal weight.
b. mortal weight.
c. desirable weight.
d. average weight.

d   7/V3   8.

Desirable weight might be defined as that weight which
a. is not associated with hypertension, diabetes, or heart disease.
b. is associated with the lowest mortality (death) rate.
c. can be maintained for more than 5 years.
d. a and b.

c   7/V3   9. Which of the following statements might be good advice from someone who has gone through many weight changes over a lifetime?
          a.   "Keep trying to change your body image - it can only get better."
          b.   "Look to fashion models as your role model - they are where it's at."
          c.   "Make peace with your body - every body type is beautiful."
          d.   "Don't worry about your health as long as you look good in clothes."

c   10/V4   10. In studies performed on women who were able to maintain their lost weight, findings showed that
          a.   they attended regular support groups.
          b.   they kept regular track of food intake.
          c.   all of them exercised regularly.
          d.   all of the above.

d   10/V4   11. The biggest factor associated with weight loss in people who managed to lose weight and keep it off was
          a.   keeping food diaries.
          b.   going to support groups.
          c.   visiting with a dietitian.
          d.   exercising on a regular basis.

a   5/V5   12. A factor in weight gain or inability to lose weight might be
          a.   a slower metabolic rate than normal for height and weight.
          b.   an increased thermogenic rate than normal for height.
          c.   the inability to increase dynamic effect of food.
          d.   any of the above.

a   5/V5   13. If people are trying to lose weight and are 20% below their predicted metabolic rate, they will
          a.   have a harder time burning kcalories and not lose much weight.
          b.   be tired most of the time and gain weight quickly.
          c.   expect to lose weight quickly on 1500 kcal/day.
          d.   a and b.

Lesson 11: Weight Control: Health Effects

Ans	Objective		
c	8/V1	1.	Compared to average weight for women in the U.S., fashion models are

c   8/V1

1. Compared to average weight for women in the U.S., fashion models are
   a. 10% below the average.
   b. 18% below the average.
   c. 23% below the average.
   d. 35% below the average.

b   8/V1

2. When comparing fashion models to the average woman in the U.S., models have body weights that are
   a. considered the ideal by the medical profession.
   b. unrealistic and unattainable for most women.
   c. attainable for most women if they work hard to lose weight.
   d. usually too high for the average height of models.

d   4/V2

3. Which of the following factors do experts consider a criterion for successful weight loss?
   a. If blood pressure went down
   b. If diabetes improved
   c. If some, but not necessarily all, weight was lost
   d. Any of the above

c   4/V2

4. If people need to lose 50 pounds of weight and only achieve a 25 pound weight loss, the criteria established by the medical profession would consider those people to be
   a. underachievers.
   b. failures.
   c. successful.
   d. hopeless.

b   9/V3

5. Total body fat or scale weight does not provide as clear an index of risk for disease as can be provided by
   a. body mass index.
   b. waist-to-hip ratio.
   c. lower body fat index.
   d. none of the above.

a   9/V3

6. People with high waist-to-hip ratios have a higher risk for heart disease and are characterized by shape as
   a. "apples."
   b. "slugs."
   c. "pears."
   d. "sloths."

d   3/V4

7. As a way to lose weight, "yo-yo" diets may produce quick weight loss
   a. with a subsequent higher regain of weight.
   b. but no permanent weight lost.
   c. and may result in a slower metabolic rate.
   d. all of the above.

c   3/V4   8. A cycle of quick weight loss and weight regain which may cause the body's metabolism to slow down is known as
   a. "cyclic regaining."
   b. "dieting madness."
   c. "yo-yo dieting."
   d. "on-off cycling."

c   2/V5   9. For people who are considered morbidly obese by medical standards, an extreme procedure in which the stomach size is restricted surgically is known as
   a. esophageal stapling.
   b. gastric liposuction.
   c. gastric bypass.
   d. divisional resection.

a   2/V5   10. An extreme surgical procedure, such as a gastric bypass, produces dramatic weight loss in morbidly obese people by
   a. restricting the size of the stomach so it holds less food.
   b. stimulating the hypothalamus to not respond to excess food.
   c. shortening the GI tract so that food is not absorbed.
   d. reducing the length of the colon so food passes quickly.

b   7/V6   11. Of the most common eating disorders, the one which is most medically dangerous is
   a. bulimia nervosa.
   b. anorexia nervosa.
   c. obesity nervosa.
   d. purging nervosa.

b   7/V6   12. One of the criteria for diagnosing anorexia is
   a. refusal to eat complex carbohydrates.
   b. being 85% or less of normal body weight for age.
   c. people see themselves as physically fit.
   d. all of the above.

d   7/V6   13. A distinguishing characteristic of people with bulimia is they
   a. eat high-protein foods without realizing it.
   b. are preoccupied with body weight and shape.
   c. believe that weight and shape are central to self-concept.
   d. b and c.

c   7/V6   14. All of the following are acceptable treatments for bulimia EXCEPT
   a. helping the person normalize eating patterns.
   b. focusing on the person's social world.
   c. treating all people with bulimia in a hospital setting.
   d. changing the attitudes regarding weight and shape.

d   4/V7   15. For a number of decades, experts have been saying that the best weight loss program involves
   a. regular exercise.
   b. eating healthful diets.
   c. keeping tract of kcalories in vs. kcalories out.
   d. all of the above.

c   4/V7   16. The best advice regarding weight gain and pregnancy is
  a. lose weight as fast as possible after pregnancy.
  b. don't gain any weight during pregnancy.
  c. lose weight slowly to keep it off permanently.
  d. eat a lot, exercise a lot, then lose a lot.

b   4/V7   17. If a woman gains as much as 45 pounds during pregnancy, the best advice regarding weight loss after pregnancy is
  a. lose weight quickly for permanent weight loss.
  b. lose weight slowly for permanent weight loss.
  c. exercise more often than before pregnancy.
  d. b and c.

Lesson 12: Vitamins: Water-Soluble

b   2/V1   1.   In which of the following ways do B vitamins interact with energy-yielding foods?
                           a.   They provide an essential source of additional energy.
                           b.   They are not a source of energy, but they are needed to convert the foods we eat into energy.
                           c.   B vitamins only interact with fatty acids to produce energy.
                           d.   B vitamins only interact with carbohydrates to produce energy.

d   5/V2   2.   Researchers state that the immune system is positively affected by
                           a.   fat-soluble vitamins.
                           b.   niacin.
                           c.   thiamin.
                           d.   vitamin C.

d   7/V3   3.   One way to manage fruits and vegetables on long voyages at sea is to
                           a.   store them in a freezer.
                           b.   replenish them in port.
                           c.   use canned products.
                           d.   all of the above.

b   7/V3   4.   As far as cooking vegetables is concerned, the key in preventing vitamin losses is to
                           a.   cook until soft to the touch.
                           b.   not overcook--keep slightly crisp.
                           c.   use a lot of water when cooking.
                           d.   drink the water in which the vegetables were cooked.

d   7/V3   5.   Much of the vitamin content in vegetables will be destroyed if they are cooked
                           a.   at high temperatures.
                           b.   for extended periods.
                           c.   submerged in water.
                           d.   all of the above.

d   7/V3   6.   Preferred ways to cook vegetables include
                           a.   steamed with a little water.
                           b.   boiled.
                           c.   microwaved.
                           d.   a and c.

Objective

2/V1   7.   What group of nutrients help to extract the energy from food during metabolism?

5/V2   8.   When studying allergies and aging, what water-soluble vitamin has been shown to have a positive effect?

Answer

7.   B vitamins (coenzymes)

8.   Vitamin C

Lesson 13: Vitamins: Fat-Soluble

<u>Ans</u>	<u>Objective</u>	

a   2/V1

1. If taken in excess, vitamin A can produce adverse effects, such as
   a. intracranial pressure in the brain resulting in headaches.
   b. blurred vision resulting in headaches.
   c. bone mineralization resulting in rickets.
   d. all of the above.

a   2/V1

2. Intracranial pressure resulting in headaches is a side effect of taking excessive amounts of vitamin
   a. A.
   b. D.
   c. E.
   d. K.

c   3/V2

3. Examples of the adverse effects of oxidation reactions include
   a. headaches brought on by vitamin A toxicity.
   b. bubbles forming when soap mixes with greasy dishes.
   c. butter or oil turning rancid or having off-flavors.
   d. all of the above.

a   3/V2

4. Rust forming on a metal surface or butter turning rancid are examples of
   a. an oxidation reaction which produces undesirable results.
   b. a mineral interacting with a hard surface.
   c. iron particles interacting with water molecules.
   d. b and c.

b   3/V3

5. Which vitamin can protect lipids, especially vitamin A and polyunsaturated fatty acids, against the effects of free radical attack?
   a. Vitamin C
   b. Vitamin E
   c. Vitamin D
   d. Vitamin K

a   3/V3

6. Several conditions and/or chronic diseases might be prevented in the future through the use of
   a. antioxidant supplementation with vitamins C and E.
   b. medications that have yet to be discovered.
   c. new exercise equipment that is currently being developed.
   d. all of the above.

b   3/V3

7. Young patients who have heart disease might be advised to take
   a. vitamin A supplements.
   b. vitamin E supplements.
   c. vitamin D supplements.
   d. multiple vitamins.

a   4/V4

8. People who participate in vigorous aerobic-type exercise could possibly benefit from vitamin C and E supplementation to prevent against
   a. tissue damage due to free radical production.
   b. muscle aches and pains associated with vigorous exercise.
   c. heart problems associated with aerobic-type exercises.
   d. the onset of heart disease which occurs when people train for marathons.

b   4/V4   9. Vitamin E supplements are often taken by runners to help prevent damage to lungs caused by

              a. heavy exercise during cold weather.
              b. exercising when air pollution is high.
              c. exercising indoors.
              d. any of the above.

d   4/V4   10. According to research, the body system, especially in the elderly, that shows improvement when given antioxidant supplements is the

              a. nervous system.
              b. respiratory system.
              c. digestive system.
              d. immune system.

Objective

2/V1   11. Excessive intakes of vitamin A have been shown to produce intracranial pressure resulting in

3/V2   12. When rust forms on an iron railing or cooking oil smells rancid, the undesirable effect is caused by a process known as

3/V3   13. When oxygen breaks down fatty acids used by the cells to produce energy for the body, potentially damaging intermediates may be produced from a process known as

4/V4   14. What body system appears to improve when elderly people take vitamin E and other antioxidants?

              Answer
              11. headaches.

              12. oxidation (free radical production).

              13. lipid peroxidation.

              14. The immune system (immunity, immune response)

Lesson 14: Major Minerals and Water

<u>Ans</u>	<u>Objective</u>	

c 8/V1

1. What percent of water loss from the body could result in a life-threatening situation?
   a. 1%
   b. 5%
   c. 10%
   d. 3%

d 8/V1

2. The very first reliable sign of dehydration is
   a. thirst.
   b. chills.
   c. cramps.
   d. fatigue.

d 8/V1

3. Some of the physical symptoms reflecting dehydration in a child might include
   a. deep, dark circles under the eyes.
   b. increased heart rate for age.
   c. dry, tacky mucous membranes in the mouth.
   d. all of the above.

d 8/V1

4. Advice to parents of a child who is dehydrated would include
   a. offering the child a teaspoon of clear liquids every 5-10 minutes.
   b. ignoring the situation until the child asks for something to drink.
   c. encouraging the child to drink liquids frequently, especially if they have been vomiting.
   d. a and c.

c 7/V2

5. Regarding sodium intake, an average adult only needs
   a. 5 grams/day or 1 teaspoon.
   b. 5000 milligrams/day or 1 teaspoon.
   c. 500 milligrams/day or 1/10 of a teaspoon.
   d. a and b.

c 9/V3

6. The population most affected by bone loss resulting in osteoporosis is
   a. males over the age of 65.
   b. female athletes who compete in marathons.
   c. women over the age of 50.
   d. all of the above in equal proportions.

a 9/V3

7. The most common cause(s) of osteoporosis is(are)
   a. lack of estrogen in postmenopausal women.
   b. increased bone formation in the elderly.
   c. lack of weight-bearing exercise during the growing years.
   d. all of the above.

a 9/V3

8. What type of exercise can improve the outcome of osteoporosis?
   a. Weight-bearing exercises, such as walking
   b. Swimming laps or water aerobics
   c. Meditation exercises
   d. All of the above

d	9/V3	9. Dietary interventions to improve osteoporosis include
		    a. increased calcium intakes.
		    b. avoidance of meat and poultry.
		    c. decreased salt intakes.
		    d. all of the above.

c	9/V3	10. The only oral medication known to stimulate bone formation and growth in patients with osteoporosis is
		    a. hypoglycemic medication.
		    b. oral insulin.
		    c. calcium citrate with slow release fluoride.
		    d. calcium gluconate with phosphorus.

d	9/V3	11. Osteoporosis can be prevented by practicing the following advice:
		    a. stop smoking.
		    b. begin early administration of estrogen.
		    c. take optimal amounts of calcium.
		    d. all of the above.

c	9/V3	12. Very often the first symptom that a person has osteoporosis is
		    a. a feeling of tenderness in the hips.
		    b. lower back problems.
		    c. a broken hip or wrist.
		    d. numbness of the toes.

a	6/V4	13. An effect of increased water intake on the body of a person who is accustomed to greater quantities of salt is
		    a. reduced edema or swelling of ankles.
		    b. more bloating.
		    c. more energy.
		    d. all of the above.

Objective

8/V1	14.	If athletes exercise for an hour, they could lose water equal to how many pounds of body weight?
8/V1	15.	Fatigue is the first reliable sign that a person is
8/V1	16.	Deep, dark circles under the eyes; lethargy; increased heart rate for age; and a dry mouth are all signs of
9/V3	17.	A slow and steady loss of bone calcium resulting in fracturing or splintering of bones is a characteristic of
9/V3	18.	Of the 25 million people with osteoporosis, what segment of the population is most affected and at what age?
9/V3	19.	The best exercise for someone with osteoporosis is
6/V4	20.	People could reduce the edema that accompanies high salt intakes by increasing their intake of

Answer

14. 2-4 pounds

15. dehydrated.

16. dehydration.

17. osteoporosis.

18. Women over 50

19. weight bearing (walking, weight training).

20. water.

Objective

9/V3   21. Discuss osteoporosis including a definition; how it develops; how age, sex, hormones, and genetics affect it; how activity affects it; and what dietary interventions can help prevent or treat osteoporosis.

Answer Explanation:

21. Answers could include the following information:

Definition: osteoporosis is a condition whereby bone density is lost, thus creating fractures.

* Development and dietary influences:
* Strongest predictor of bone density is age, followed by sex.
* Skeletal growth and density occurs during the first two and a half decades of life.
* Calcium absorption declines after about age 65.
* Vitamin D is less active after age 65, therefore less calcium absorption.
* Women suffer from osteoporosis more than men before age 75, then it equals in frequency.
* Estrogen as well as testosterone play a part in the development of osteoporosis, but estrogen seems to be more protective in women up to menopause.
* Asian and Caucasian women have more osteoporosis than other ethnic groups.
* Weight bearing activities are protective against osteoporosis.
* High protein intakes seem to promote calcium excretion, thereby decreasing bone density.
* Dietary calcium and/or calcium supplements are necessary to maintain bone density as well as possibly fluoride supplements.

Lesson 15: Trace Minerals

<u>Ans</u>	<u>Objective</u>	

d   4/V1   1. The population(s) at greatest risk for iron deficiency is(are)
   a. low-income, pregnant women.
   b. low-income children.
   c. adult males.
   d. a and b.

b   4/V1   2. What is the major cause of iron deficiency?
   a. Blood loss
   b. Poor nutrition
   c. Hereditary defect
   d. Parasitic infections of the GI tract

c   2/V1   3. Nonheme iron absorption can be enhanced by
   a. tea.
   b. coffee.
   c. foods containing vitamin C.
   d. food containing vitamin E.

d   1/V4   4. What iron-containing compound carries oxygen in the bloodstream?
   a. Ferritin
   b. myoglobin
   c. transferring
   d. hemoglobin

b   2/V1   5. Absorption of iron from supplements is improved by taking them with
   a. tea.
   b. meat.
   c. milk.
   d. whole grain bread.

c   4/V2   6. Signs of iron toxicity include all of the following EXCEPT
   a. apathy.
   b. fatigue.
   c. hypochromic anemia.
   d. increases in infections.

c   4/V2   7. Which of the following disorders is positively correlated with the presence of high blood iron?
   a. Dermatitis
   b. Diverticulosis
   c. Heart Disease
   d. Neural tube defects

b	4/V2	8.	The most common cause of iron overload is

8. The most common cause of iron overload is
   a. an injury to the GI tract.
   b. a genetic predisposition.
   c. excessive use of iron cookware.
   d. excessive use of iron supplements.

a   9/V4

9. What is the most reliable source of dietary fluoride?
   a. Public water
   b. Dark green vegetables
   c. Milk and milk products
   d. Meats and whole grain cereals

a   9/V4

10. Fluoride deficiency is best known to lead to
    a. dental decay.
    b. osteoporosis.
    c. discoloration of teeth.
    d. nutritional muscular dystrophy.

C   9/V3

11. One of the chief functions of chromium is participation in the metabolism of
    a. iron.
    b. proteins.
    c. carbohydrates.
    d. metallothionein.

b   9/V3

12. In some studies, what population may benefit from chromium supplements?
    a. People wanting to build muscle mass
    b. People with diabetes
    c. People who are vegetarians
    d. People with high cholesterol

C   11/V5

13. What term designates foods that contain nonnutrient substances which may provide health benefits beyond basic nutrition?
    a. Health foods
    b. Organic foods
    c. Functional foods
    d. Disease preventative foods

c   11/V5

14. What phytochemical is present in tomato-based products?
    a. Limonene
    b. Tannins
    c. Lycopene
    d. Indoles

d   5/V6

15. By replacing meat sources of iron in the diet with plant sources of iron, someone with a high risk for heart disease would also
    a. be reducing the nonheme form of iron which is most easily absorbed, therefore decreasing risk for heart disease.
    b. be reducing the heme form of iron which is most easily absorbed, therefore decreasing risk for heart disease.
    c. be reducing saturated fat in the diet, therefore decreasing risk for heart disease.
    d. b and c.

1/V1   16.   What is the most important mineral for growth and development in infants?

2/V1   17.   What is the name of the substance found in plant foods that can bind with iron or zinc and render them unavailable for absorption?

2/V5   18.   Replacing meat sources of iron with plant sources could reduce the risk for heart disease while automatically reducing iron intake in the form of

Answer

16.   Iron

17.   Phytate (phytic acid)

18.   heme iron.

Lesson 16: Physical Activity: Fitness Basics

Ans	Objective		
b	1/V1	1.	Research clearly shows that the risk of dying not only from heart disease but from all causes is greatest for

b   1/V1   1. Research clearly shows that the risk of dying not only from heart disease but from all causes is greatest for
   a. elite athletes such as marathoners.
   b. sedentary people, a.k.a. "couch potatoes."
   c. occasional exercisers, a.k.a. "week-end warriors."
   d. moderately active people who exercise 3-4 days/week.

a   1/V1   2. Research has shown that being sedentary
   a. increases the risk of dying from all causes.
   b. is better than being sporadically active.
   c. is not harmful as long as the person makes wise nutrition choices.
   d. can actually help a person who has suffered from a heart attack.

d   1/V2   3. Overexercising has its drawback for those who try to do too much because it
   a. may increase the risk for type II diabetes in some people.
   b. can cause muscle injuries that only rest and time will heal.
   c. can frustrate people if they do not see real improvements in performance.
   d. may compromise the immune system and may ultimately lead to diseases such as cancer.

c   1/V2   4. Individuals who run 60 or 70 miles/week, such as marathon runners, may actually
   a. feel it is not enough to achieve their goals.
   b. be overexercising to the benefit of their health.
   c. suppress their immune function and cause disease.
   d. all of the above.

d   5/V3   5. In addition to being able to exercise at work, employees who have access to a Wellness program and fitness facility at the job site
   a. is more likely to make positive changes in lifestyle.
   b. has less absenteeism from work.
   c. becomes more educated in health issues.
   d. all of the above.

b   8/V3   6. Among the physiological benefits of regular exercise, which of the following can occur?
   a. Regular exercise will inhibit the blood chemistry responsible for the "good" cholesterol.
   b. Regular exercise can be a way to improve mood and relieve depression.
   c. Regular exercise has been shown to increase the need for "energizers."
   d. Regular exercise decreases blood flow to the brain, therefore activating endorphins, natural tranquilizers.

d   8/V3   7. Some companies use a Wellness program or fitness facility as a vehicle to
   a. recruit employees.
   b. increase morale of employees.
   c. control employee exercise programs.
   d. A and B.

146

c   8/V4   8. The general recommendation to support activity is to eat a diet
     a. high in protein and low in fat.
     b. low in protein and high in carbohydrate.
     c. high in carbohydrate and low in fat.
     d. high in carbohydrate and high in protein.

c   8/V4   9. Regardless of the intensity of an exercise program, the best diet emphasizes
     a. protein.
     b. fat.
     c. carbohydrate.
     d. water.

a   8/V4,V5   10. The very best combination of diet and exercise for an individual who is interested in achieving the basic elements of health is
     a. lots of complex carbohydrates and regular exercise regardless of the intensity.
     b. exercise two times a week with occasional "junk" food treats.
     c. moderate amounts of meat and fried foods combined with weight training two times a week.
     d. regular consumption of sports drinks and vigorous exercise at least three times a week.

d   8/V5   11. Walking is considered the best form of exercise because it
     a. is not expensive.
     b. promotes cardiovascular endurance.
     c. is easy to perform.
     d. all of the above.

c   8/V5   12. The most important component(s) of exercise from a health and longevity standpoint is(are)
     a. the intensity and duration of the activity.
     b. the duration and frequency of the activity.
     c. the frequency and regularity of the activity.
     d. the warm-up and cool-down periods.

c   8/V6   13. Before undertaking an exercise or nutrition program, what preliminary steps should be taken?
     a. Choose an expensive activity; that way you know you've invested money in it and be more likely to stay with it.
     b. Go to an exercise physiologist who can teach you how the body works.
     c. Choose an enjoyable activity that you know you will stay with whether you're alone or in a group.
     d. Get an exercise stress test from a sports medicine doctor who is also knowledgeable in nutrition.

a   8/V6   14. A person with high blood cholesterol should consider participating in an aerobic exercise program such as walking or jogging because aerobic exercise
　　　　　　　　　　　　　　　a. will raise HDL ("good") cholesterol after a period of training and decrease the risk for heart disease.
　　　　　　　　　　　　　　　b. will cause a sudden increase in the heartrate to near maximal levels which lowers the "bad" cholesterol.
　　　　　　　　　　　　　　　c. forces more LDL ("bad") cholesterol out of the body through waste elimination.
　　　　　　　　　　　　　　　d. keeps the blood circulating faster, even at rest, therefore causes a decrease in total blood cholesterol.

Objective

1/V1   15. According to research, what population has an increased risk of dying of heart attack or any other cause?

5/V3   16. What type of exercise has been shown to reduce depression due to a release of brain endorphins?

Answer

15. Sedentary people

16. Aerobic exercise

Lesson 17: Physical Activity: Beyond Fitness

Ans	Objective		
a	2/V1	1.	By eating a high carbohydrate diet the day before any athletic event, a. muscles will have adequate fuel, i.e., glycogen for the competition. b. athletes can eat more protein the day of the competition. c. less water will be needed the day of the competition since carbohydrates are high in water. d. all of the above.
d	7/V1	2.	Regardless of the physical pursuits of an athlete, the recommended diet should be a foundation of a. protein. b. amino acids. c. water. d. complex carbohydrates.
d	7/V1	3.	On the day of a competition, athletes should eat a. enough to feel "fed" but not "full." b. enough food to keep their blood sugar levels up. c. complex carbohydrates and plenty of fluids. d. all of the above.
d	7/V1	4.	If athletes are going to drink caffeinated beverages prior to competition, they a. should first try it out in practice to make sure it doesn't produce adverse side effects. b. need to experiment during training to see if it helps make the exercise seem easier. c. should drink them at least four hours before the event. d. a and b.
c	7/V2	5.	What dietary components might athletes in wheelchairs need less of and more of, respectively, than other athletes? a. Protein and carbohydrates b. Fat and protein c. kCalories and water d. Vitamins and minerals
b	9/V2	6.	Physical activity is very important for physically challenged people because a. it keeps them from becoming bored. b. they can eat more and, by consuming more nutrients, become healthier. c. they are not as strong as people who are not physically challenged. d. all of the above.
d	9/V2	7.	Exercise and nutrition are important components of a sound program for physically challenged people because they a. are investments in good physical health. b. help support a positive mental health. c. help people face the challenges of life and achieve dreams. d. all of the above.

c   8/V3   8. For most athletes who are well-nourished, nutrition supplements such as protein powders and vitamin pills
   a. dramatically improve performance.
   b. improve performance only moderately.
   c. do not significantly improve performance.
   d. seem to cause a decrease in performance.

d   8/V3   9. There is evidence that athletes who have taken steroids for as few as five years have developed
   a. blood cysts in the liver.
   b. cancer of the liver.
   c. impotence in males.
   d. all of the above.

d   8/V3   10. A proven ergogenic aid that helps endurance athletes achieve a boost in energy is
   a. water.
   b. coffee.
   c. chocolate.
   d. sports drinks.

d   9/V4   11. It has been demonstrated that regular aerobic exercise will help
   a. improve energy levels.
   b. reduce stress.
   c. improve HDL levels.
   d. all of the above.

Objective

2/V1   12. The substance that is most depleted during repetitive type exercises is

7/V1   13. The foundation of an athlete's diet should consist of

8/V3   14. Epoetin, steroids, and blood doping, all of which have been touted to improve athletic performance, are examples of

9/V4   15. Regular aerobic exercise has been shown to improve which components of a blood lipid profile?

Answer

12. muscle glycogen

13. complex carbohydrates

14. ergogenic aids.

15. HDL (or triglycerides)

Lesson 18: Life Cycle: Pregnancy

Ans	Objective	Q#	
d	5/V1	01.	Advice to pregnant women who want to exercise includes a. don't begin a new program. b. swim, but do not lift weights c. walk, but not too intensely. d. all of the above.
a	5/V1	02.	Swimming is actually one of the best exercises for a. placental blood profusion. b. losing weight while pregnant. c. increasing abdominal strength. d. increasing stress to the fetus.
c	4/V2	03.	What percent of weight gain during pregnancy is due to maternal fat weight? a. 15% b. 20% c. 30% d. 45%
b	4/V2	04.	Dieting during pregnancy is a. recommended if the mother is overweight. b. not recommended at all. c. dependant upon the initial weight of the mother. d. directly correlated to high birthweight.
c	11/V3	05.	The highest at-risk age for pregnancy is a. 6-years postmenarchy. b. 4-years postmenarchy. c. 2-years postmenarchy. d. none of the above.
a	11/V3	06.	The risk associated with teenage pregnancy is a a. low-birthweight infant. b. high-birthweight infant. c. low incidence of miscarriage. d. high incidence of gestational diabetes.
d	11/V3	07.	The recommendation for iron supplementation is a. greater for pregnant teens. b. about 30-60 milligrams/day. c. necessary to preserve iron stores. d. all of the above.
d	11/V3	08.	The recommendation for folic acid is a. about 400 micrograms/day. b. necessary to prevent neural tube defects. c. lower than the RDA. d. a and b.
c	11/V3	09.	Supplementation of folic acid is known to prevent a. eclampsia in pregnant women. b. gestational diabetes in pregnant women. c. spina bifida and other neural tube defects. d. pregnancy-induced hypertension.

d   13/V4   10.   Among the reasons young mothers lose sight of personal fitness or nutrition goals is
      a.   overwork and fatigue.
      b.   stresses of being a new mother.
      c.   post-partum depression.
      d.   all of the above.

b   13/V4   11.   A young mother can reach personal fitness and nutrition goals by
      a.   asking her doctor for a tranquilizer.
      b.   finding a comfortable way to work through changes.
      c.   spending more time working out at a gym.
      d.   eating foods that are low-fat.

Lesson 19: Life Cycle: Lactation and Infancy

a   7/V1

1. Research has shown that breastfed infants probably need
   a. fewer kcalories than formula fed infants.
   b. more kcalories than formula fed infants.
   c. more iron than formula fed infants.
   d. less iron than formula fed infants.

a   7/V1

2. Compared to formula fed infants, breast fed infants seem to need
   a. less energy.
   b. more energy.
   c. more iron.
   d. less iron.

d   7/V2

3. Indications that an infant is getting enough food are
   a. six to eight wet diapers/day.
   b. one bowel movement/day.
   c. infant is alert and happy.
   d. any of the above.

a   7/V2

4. One of the ways you can tell if an infant is getting enough food is
   a. by the number of wet diapers/day.
   b. if the infant is gaining two lbs./week.
   c. if the infant sleeps through the night by three weeks of age.
   d. by the number of feedings/day.

a   5/V3

5. A woman who is not breastfeeding
   a. has the same nutrient requirements as non-lactating women.
   b. needs more nutrients than non-lactating women.
   c. has the same nutrient requirements as lactating women.
   d. has a greater need for water than lactating women.

b   7/V3

6. Compared to breast feeding women, formula feeding women
   a. have identical nutrient needs.
   b. have fewer nutrient needs.
   c. need more water.
   d. need less water.

b   7/V4

7. Nutrition scientists agree that cow's milk can be given to infants
   a. as soon as they can sit up.
   b. after the age of 12 months.
   c. who are eating solid foods.
   d. any of the above.

c   7/V4

8. The recommended age to introduce cow's milk to infants is
   a. four to six months.
   b. six to 12 months.
   c. after 12 months.
   d. after two years.

b   7/V4

9. Breastfed infants need an additional iron source
   a. after they've been weaned.
   b. at about six months.
   c. at three months.
   d. they don't - they get enough iron from breast milk.

c   7/V5   10.   Some research shows that introducing fruits before vegetables
           a.   will cause the infant to develop a sweet tooth.
           b.   causes more allergic reactions.
           c.   has little impact on future food preferences.
           d.   causes excess weight gain in the infant.

a   7/V5   11.   The recommended order of introducing fruits and vegetables to infants
           a.   doesn't seem to matter.
           b.   is fruits then vegetables.
           c.   is vegetables then fruits.
           d.   is to mix them together at the same meal.

c   10/V6   12.   Stress in the mother who breastfeeds has been shown to
           a.   inhibit the quality of milk produced.
           b.   cause greater milk production.
           c.   inhibit the let-down reflex.
           d.   cause weight loss in the infant.

d   10/V6   13.   The let-down reflex
           a.   triggers the release of milk from the breasts.
           b.   can be inhibited by physical or emotional stress.
           c.   occurs after the baby is born and is temporary.
           d.   a and b.

Objective

7/V2   14.   Cite one guideline to determine if an infant is getting enough food.

7/V4   15.   Cow's milk can be given after what age?

Answer

14.   May include any of the following:
     * 6-8 wet diapers/day
     * One bowel movement/day
     * Happy and alert baby
     * Appropriate weight gain

15.   12 months (one year)

Lesson 20: Life Cycle: Childhood and Adolescence

Ans	Objective	

Ans   **Objective**

b   4/V1   1. The first concrete element associated with trust, safety, and security between an infant and the primary caregiver is
   a. love.
   b. food.
   c. attention.
   d. all of the above.

a   4/V1   2. When food is overly important or not attended to properly in the family, experts have found that there
   a. are more eating disorders.
   b. are fewer incidences of binging and purging.
   c. is a greater chance for discipline problems.
   d. all of the above.

b   4/V1   3. With regard to food intake, if parents do not set limits for children, children will
   a. probably become obese by the time they are adolescents.
   b. not learn to set limits for themselves in other aspects of life as well.
   c. become too independent as adults.
   d. all of the above.

d   5/V2   4. Parents can teach children to become responsible with regard to food intake by
   a. modeling the behavior they want the children to learn.
   b. creating positive learning experiences around food.
   c. giving children a certain amount of authority with regard to food choices.
   d. all of the above.

a   5/V2   5. An example of a parent giving children appropriate authority with regard to food intake might be
   a. allowing a four-year-old to choose a snack from a banana or whole wheat bread.
   b. telling a 16-year-old to eat all his meal before having dessert.
   c. begging an 18-year-old to eat homemade bean soup for dinner.
   d. allowing a six-year-old to go grocery shopping alone.

c   5/V3   6. If parents habitually overeat past the point of satiety, children will learn to
   a. disregard their parents' actions and learn to eat sensibly.
   b. listen to their own bodies and respond appropriately to internal hunger cues.
   c. disregard their own internal hunger and satiety cues and habitually overeat.
   d. listen to their peers when it comes to eating appropriately.

a   5/V3   7. Children will learn to disregard their own internal hunger and satiety cues if they
   a. observe their parents habitually overeating.
   b. watch too much television, especially food advertisements.
   c. eat too many complex carbohydrates during the day.
   d. drink too many soft drinks.

d	5/V4	8.	The weight loss program known as ShapeDown helps adolescents lose excess weight by

d   5/V4   8. The weight loss program known as ShapeDown helps adolescents lose excess weight by
   a. treating not only the body but also the mind.
   b. utilizing an interdisciplinary team of professionals.
   c. involving all family members in the program.
   d. all of the above.

d   5/V4   9. The most powerful factor(s) to impact adolescent weight loss include(s)
   a. genetics.
   b. the closeness of the family.
   c. peers.
   d. a and b.

a   9/V5   10. Adolescent girls who believe they do not measure up to media portrayal of the perfect young body image
   a. may develop eating disorders.
   b. develop a stronger self-image and more confidence.
   c. usually are more accepting of their bodies in spite of the magazines.
   d. frequently commit suicide.

d   9/V5   11. Teen magazines could have a positive influence on adolescent body-image and self-image if the magazines would
   a. focus on things teens can do rather than on what teens look like.
   b. show "real" teens of all ethnic backgrounds and shapes and not teen models.
   c. not emphasize the "Barbie" doll look as the ideal for teens.
   d. all of the above.

b   7/V6   12. Experts agree that people with type II diabetes who ate foods high in fat or sugar as adolescents
   a. developed the disease because of their eating habits.
   b. developed the disease because of their genetic background.
   c. developed the disease because they were obese to begin with.
   d. all of the above.

a   7/V6   13. Adolescents who snack on high-fat foods or sugary foods will develop type II diabetes as adults if they
   a. are genetically predisposed.
   b. do not change their eating habits.
   c. gain too much weight.
   d. all of the above.

Lesson 21: Life Cycle: Adulthood and Aging

<u>Answer</u>	<u>Objective</u>		
d	4/V1	1.	Relative to muscle mass, which of the following nutrients should be decreased? a. Fat b. High kcalorie foods c. Total kcalories d. All of the above
d	8/V2	2	Scientists are trying to convince older people a. that it's not how long we live, but how successfully. b. to stop trying to grow old gracefully. c. that it's best to go out like a light bulb-bright and quick!. d. a and c.
b	8/V2	3.	If scientists had their way, when it was time to die, we all should a. spend our remaining years in bed! b. go quickly, like a light bulb! c. be glad that medical science prolonged our life even in the absence of quality. d. none of the above.
d	5/V3	4.	Exercises that help prevent the age-related decrease in muscle mass a. are non-existent. b. should include light weight training. c. can be as simple as regular daily walking. d. b and c.
d	9/V4	5.	Alcohol use is not recommended for the elderly because a. blood alcohol levels rise more quickly. b. they have less body water due to less muscle mass. c. they are more sensitive to alcohol's effects. d. all of the above.
d	9/V4	6.	Alcohol can affect an older adult a. by increasing blood alcohol level quickly. b. because they are more sensitive to alcohol's effects. c. because they have less body water to dilute it. d. all of the above.
a	7/V5	7.	Diabetes impacts aging in which of the following ways? a. If blood glucose level is not well controlled, a person could die earlier than expected. b. A person with diabetes usually won't live beyond age 65. c. Diabetes is associated with liver damage, therefore shorter life span. d. Diabetes can't impact longevity, especially if there is no heredity factor.
d	7/V5	8.	A person who has lived with diabetes for 20 - 40 years a. is more likely to have complications associated with the disease. b. is not likely to suffer any more ill effects than a younger person with the disease. c. should pay especially close attention to the level of glycemic control. d. a and c.

Objective

4/V1	9.	As you age there is less of a need for foods that are high in
5/V3	10.	As a person ages there is a relative loss of
5/V3	11.	The type of exercise recommended to prevent osteoporosis is

Objective   **Answer**

9. kcalories (fat, energy).

10. muscle mass (lean body mass, muscle strength).

11. weight bearing (walking, jogging, weight lifting, dancing, etc.).

Lesson 22: Diet and Health: Cardiovascular Disease

Ans	Objective		
c	4/V1	1.	The single MOST preventable risk factor associated with cardiac disease and stroke is a. obesity. b. alcohol. c. smoking. d. heredity.
d	6/V1	2.	High blood pressure (hypertension) is caused by a. obesity. b. smoking. c. lack of exercise. d. all of the above.
d	6/V1	3.	High blood pressure or hypertension causes physical damage to the blood vessel walls and results in a. the formation of plaque. b. heart disease. c. stroke. d. all of the above.
b	4/V1	4.	On the average and compared to men, women tend to get heart disease a. as frequently as men. b. about 7-10 years later than men. c. but have fewer complications than men. d. all of the above.
a	5/V1	5.	As researchers found out more about blood cholesterol, the recommended acceptable value for blood cholesterol has a. dropped from 260 mg/dl to less than 200 mg/dl in a decade. b. steadily increased up to 200 mg/dl in the past decade. c. remained the same for 25 years. d. only reflected LDL values.
b	3/V1	6.	Part of the protection against heart disease women enjoy seems to come from the fact that women a. are generally less stressed out than men. b. produce estrogen which is known to elevate HDL and protect them. c. have generally lower total cholesterol than men. d. a and b.
b	4/V1	7.	Populations that may be more susceptible to potential heart damage caused by elevated triglycerides include people with a. osteoporosis. b. diabetes. c. cancer. d. AIDS.
c	2/V1	8.	A significant reduction in blood flow to the brain is termed a. angina. b. stroke. c. Vascular event. d. Metabolic syndrome.

a   5/V2   9.   In general, experts recommend that to prevent heart disease, mortality and morbidity, people should exercise
   a.   daily for 30-40 minutes at moderate pace.
   b.   every other day for 50 minutes at moderate pace.
   c.   twice a week for one hour at intense pace.
   d.   any of the above, depending on your schedule.

b   4/V2   10.   When LDL level is elevated and HDL is lower than recommended, the first thing that should be examined is a person's
   a.   alcohol intake.
   b.   exercise program.
   c.   genetic background.
   d.   smoking habits.

a   5/V2   11.   In addition to regular exercise, equally important in the prevention of heart disease is
   a.   reducing fat intake, especially saturated fat.
   b.   increasing monounsaturated fat intake.
   c.   eliminating cholesterol from the diet.
   d.   reducing the servings of dairy in the diet.

d   4/V1   12.   High blood cholesterol is generally due to
   a.   genetics.
   b.   poor diet.
   c.   lack of exercise.
   d.   all of the above.

d   8/ V2   13.   Which of the following is NOT among the recommendations by health professionals to treat hypertension?
   a.   Increase dietary fiber
   b.   Decrease sodium intake
   c.   If overweight, reduce weight
   d.   Decrease potassium intake

d   5/V2   14.   To see a significant regression in coronary disease, many experts recommend
   a.   a very low-fat diet of no more than 10% of total kcalories.
   b.   more regular aerobic exercise.
   c.   a vegetarian eating plan with no meat.
   d.   all of the above.

a   5/V2   15.   The reason why many experts recommend vegetarian diets is because they
   a.   have little, if any, dietary cholesterol.
   b.   are proven to provide protection against all diseases.
   c.   have been shown to significantly increase longevity in all populations.
   d.   all of the above.

b   5/V2   16.   A strong recommendation for people who are going through lifestyle and nutrition changes to reduce heart disease is to
   a.   grin and bear it.
   b.   be flexible and open to change.
   c.   go for it - all or nothing!
   d.   none of the above.

Lesson 23: Diet and Health: Cancer, Immunology, and AIDS

<u>Ans</u>	<u>Objective</u>	

c   3/V1

1. The type of fat that is most frequently associated with the growth of breast cancer is
   a. monounsaturated fat.
   b. saturated fat.
   c. polyunsaturated fat.
   d. vegetable fat.

b   4/V1

2. Experts suggest that the threshold of fat intake to prevent breast cancer is
   a. less than 30% of total kcalories.
   b. less than 20% of total kcalories.
   c. about 30% of total kcalories.
   d. about 45% of total kcalories.

a   4/V1

3. The American Cancer Society offers six suggestions for reducing the risk for cancer, including
   a. maintaining desirable body weight.
   b. eating the same types of foods daily.
   c. maintaining fiber intake at 10-15 grams/day.
   d. eating salt-cured foods, such as bacon, no more than three times/week.

d   4/V1

4. The American Cancer Society suggests that women and men maintain desirable weight based on the following criteria:
   a. women should weigh 100 pounds for five feet plus five pounds for each inch over five feet.
   b. both women and men should weigh 106 pounds for five feet plus six pounds for each inch over five feet.
   c. men should weigh 106 pounds for five feet plus six pounds for each inch over five feet.
   d. a and c.

a   4/V1

5. The recommendation from the American Cancer Society regarding alcohol intake and cancer prevention is to
   a. drink alcohol in limited amounts, if at all.
   b. drink an established amount of alcohol daily.
   c. become a teetotaler.
   d. consume beer or wine instead of hard liquor.

b   4/V1

6. The statement that best characterizes fiber with regard to its positive impact on the prevention of cancer is:
   a. eat soluble fiber, such as oat bran, to reduce cancer risk.
   b. eat insoluble fiber, such as wheat bran, to reduce cancer risk.
   c. eat at least 10 grams of fiber/day to reduce cancer risk.
   d. b and c.

b   4/V1

7. In addition to the fiber found in cruciferous vegetables (cabbage and broccoli), other compounds that might have a positive effect on cancers are known as
   a. oxygen-retarding agents.
   b. phytochemicals.
   c. vitamin precursors.
   d. lipid oxidizers.

d   5/V2   8. Among hospitalized patients, health professionals see a general pattern with regard to immune function in that
   a. appetite decreases and patients become malnourished.
   b. immune function improves because of overall good care.
   c. lack of nutrients leads to faulty immune function.
   d. a and c.

a   5/V2   9. Because of the lack of appetite, hospitalized patients can
   a. become malnourished resulting in poor immune function.
   b. lose unwanted body fat and unwanted pounds.
   c. become more susceptible to AIDS or cancer.
   d. all of the above.

c   5/V2   10. Elderly people are usually subjects in studies on the immune system because as they age their immune systems
   a. become stronger, allowing us to study longevity.
   b. are more likely to be resistant to unusual viruses.
   c. become the models to see how nutrition impacts immunity.
   d. have been exposed to more viruses and bacterial infections.

a   5/V2   11. By studying the immune systems of elderly people, health professionals are learning
   a. what nutrients appear promising in reducing risk of diseases such as cancer.
   b. that nutrition does not help people grow old more successfully.
   c. to turn back the hands of time by supplementing with specific nutrients.
   d. all of the above.

b   5/V2   12. All of the following are simple rules to follow to help people strengthen their immune systems EXCEPT
   a. maintain body weight within 10% of the ideal for age and sex.
   b. use supplemental fiber equal to ten grain products daily.
   c. limit dietary fat intake to less than 30% of total kcalories.
   d. eat five servings of fruits and vegetables daily.

d   5/V2   13. When recommending supplemental antioxidant vitamins/minerals for people with compromised immune systems, experts agree that
   a. people should take them in prescribed safe doses so harm will be caused.
   b. they still do not know what the appropriate doses are for this population.
   c. people should not take greater than twice the RDA for antioxidants.
   d. all of the above.

d   6/V3   14. HIV can be defined as
   a. a virus.
   b. an infection that attacks the immune system.
   c. a disease that attacks the T-4 cells in the body.
   d. all of the above.

c   6/V3   15. When CD-4 cell count is less than 200 and people have one or more opportunistic infections, they are defined as having
   a. HIV.
   b. multiple sclerosis.
   c. AIDS.
   d. Kaposi's sarcoma.

d	6/V3	16.	People with AIDS must have good nutritional support because

16. People with AIDS must have good nutritional support because
   a. malnutrition can negatively impact the immune system further.
   b. good nutrition can add years of life to the AIDS patient.
   c. they will not be able to fight opportunistic infections as well without good nutrition.
   d. all of the above.

17. Nutritional strategies that are provided to AIDS patients include
   a. nutrition education and intervention to preserve immunity.
   b. discussions on safe food handling and preparation.
   c. use of non-traditional supplements that have shown to improve immunity.
   d. a and b.

18. Non-traditional nutrition supplements such as blue-green algae or potassium drinks may
   a. help improve immune function in AIDS patients.
   b. bring about weight gain in the form of lean body mass.
   c. interfere with medications or cause toxicity.
   d. offer a safe alternative treatment for AIDS.

19. Compared to healthy people, AIDS patients require a higher intake of
   a. carbohydrate.
   b. protein.
   c. fat.
   d. vitamins.

20. The most commonly malabsorbed nutrient(s) in AIDS patients is(are)
   a. lactose or milk sugar.
   b. protein or amino acids.
   c. fatty acids.
   d. a and c.

21. Multivitamin and mineral supplements are recommended to AIDS patients because they
   a. do not absorb some nutrients.
   b. typically eat only one meal/day.
   c. eat so many sweets and fatty desserts.
   d. all of the above.

22. People who have AIDS have a recommended dietary intake based on the following nutrient breakdown:
   a. 50% carbohydrate, 30% protein, 20% fat.
   b. 40% carbohydrate, 40% protein, 20% fat.
   c. 50% carbohydrate, 50% protein, no fat.
   d. 60% carbohydrate, 35% protein, 5% fat.

23. Very high protein intakes are recommended to AIDS patients because they
   a. become anorexic and lose lean body mass.
   b. are in negative nitrogen balance due to wasting.
   c. cannot tolerate high carbohydrate foods as a rule.
   d. a and b.

The answer key and source references in the left margin are:

Answer	Reference	Question
d	6/V3	16
d	6/V3	17
c	6/V3	18
b	6/V3	19
d	6/V3	20
a	6/V3	21
b	6/V3	22
d	6/V3	23

c   6/V3   24. To prevent against the effects of anorexia, AIDS patients are encouraged to
                              a.   eat frequent large meals throughout the day.
                              b.   take medications to prevent vomiting.
                              c.   consume an instant breakfast or milkshake between meals.
                              d.   all of the above.

Lesson 24: Diet and Health: Diabetes

Ans	Objective	

d   2/V1

1. Insulin injections are required daily for people with type I diabetes because
   a. their bodies do not produce insulin.
   b. it prevents many metabolic problems from occurring.
   c. insulin stimulates the cells to remove glucose from the blood.
   d. all of the above.

a   3/V1

2. Severe weight loss, ketone production, and coma are metabolic complications generally associated with
   a. type I diabetes.
   b. type II diabetes.
   c. all diabetic conditions.
   d. hypoglycemia.

c   2/V2

3. Because onset is more gradual with type II diabetes, making diagnosis difficult, experts surmise that
   a. more than one-fourth of all people with diabetes remain undiagnosed.
   b. more than one-third of all people with diabetes remain undiagnosed.
   c. more than one-half of all people with diabetes remain undiagnosed.
   d. more than three-fourths of all people with diabetes remain undiagnosed.

d   2/V2

4. The risk factors associated with the onset of type II diabetes include
   a. having a genetic background of diabetes.
   b. being a female.
   c. being over age 40.
   d. all of the above.

b   2/V2

5. Of the following populations, the group at highest risk for type II diabetes is
   a. males under 40 years.
   b. females over 40 years.
   c. children under 11 years.
   d. adolescents between 14 and 18 years.

d   2/V3

6. When children with type I diabetes are released from the hospital, the primary role of diabetes educators is to
   a. teach parents/families how to give insulin injections.
   b. give the children their insulin injections until they are old enough to give them to themselves.
   c. teach parents how to perform blood glucose tests.
   d. a and c.

a   3/V3

7. For parents of very young children with type I diabetes, the primary responsibility of the parents is to
   a. learn to test for blood glucose levels.
   b. teach their child to give themselves insulin injections.
   c. keep children calm so they do not increase blood glucose.
   d. all of the above.

b   3/V3

8. Children with insulin-dependent diabetes should be monitored by medical professionals frequently because
   a. children frequently forget to take insulin injections.
   b. diabetes can adversely affect heart, eyes, and kidneys.
   c. parents are not willing to take responsibility for their children.
   d. all of the above.

b   4/V3

9. Sweets and desserts can be included in the diet of a child with type I diabetes as long as they are
   a. given in very small amounts only twice/week.
   b. incorporated into a diet rich in fiber and complex carbohydrates.
   c. balanced with increased amounts of protein-rich foods.
   d. all of the above.

a   5/V3

10. Care must be taken with regard to exercise in children with type I diabetes because exercise
    a. can decrease the amount of insulin needed during the day.
    b. has been shown to increase the amount of insulin needed.
    c. is not beneficial to children with type I diabetes.
    d. a and c.

d   2/V4

11. The onset of diabetes type II is associated with all of the following factors EXCEPT
    a. being female.
    b. being overweight.
    c. being over forty.
    d. being male.

b   3/V4

12. Diabetes is the number one cause of which of the following conditions/diseases?
    a. Heart disease
    b. Blindness
    c. Amputation
    d. Kidney failure

c   3/V4

13. What percent of non-accidental or non-traumatic amputations of the feet, toes, or legs is attributed to diabetes?
    a. 25%
    b. 50%
    c. 75%
    d. 100%

a   3/V4

14. What percent of new cases of end stage renal failure leading to dialysis is a consequence of diabetes?
    a. About 40%
    b. About 20%
    c. About 10%
    d. None of the above

c   3/V4   15. Of the people who die of cardiovascular disease, what percent will have diabetes as well?
   a. 50%
   b. 70%
   c. 85%
   d. 100%

c   5/V5   16. Glucose uptake can be increased by 10-20% above normal if a person with diabetes
   a. takes oral agents in addition to insulin injections.
   b. eats only foods high in complex carbohydrates and animal protein.
   c. exercises on a regular basis.
   d. all of the above.

a   5/V5   17. Exercise is encouraged early on in the treatment of diabetes because exercise can
   a. stimulate muscles to take up 10-20 times more glucose than nonexercising muscles.
   b. prevent the heart problems associated with diabetes.
   c. prevent amputations because exercising legs are stimulated to release stored glycogen.
   d. burn excess kcalories and reduce body fat associated with the onset of diabetes.

d   4/V6   18. Some medical experts state that the effects of raw vegetable diets on type II diabetes will
   a. reduce the need for insulin because people will lose significant weight on these diets.
   b. not provide all the nutrients necessary for body maintenance.
   c. need to be studied more to understand its effects on type II diabetes.
   d. all of the above.

Lesson 25: Consumer Concerns and Food Safety

Ans	Objective		

a 　 7/V1

1. What is the primary reason bottled water sales have increased dramatically over the past several years?
   a. People believe that tap water from the public water supply is unhealthy or unclean.
   b. Manufacturers of bottled water have made it inexpensive to buy when compared to tap water.
   c. Grocery stores have increased the shelf space, making bottled water more visible to consumers.
   d. All of the above.

d 　 7/V1

2. As an indication of the popularity of bottled water, sales of bottled water have surpassed the sale of
   a. milk.
   b. soft drinks.
   c. beer and wine.
   d. b and c.

b 　 7/V1

3. To determine the source of bottled water, it is always best to
   a. ask the store manager.
   b. read the label.
   c. assume it is from a spring.
   d. check with friends.

d 　 4/V2

4. Some of the alternatives to pesticide use for organic farming include
   a. earthworm castings.
   b. bat guana.
   c. seedless cow manure.
   d. all of the above.

c 　 4/V2

5. An example of an insect that can be used to repel or eat other insects that damage or destroy crops is the
   a. cockroach.
   b. June bug.
   c. lady bug.
   d. earthworm.

a 　 4/V2

6. As a way of repelling certain pests from destroying preferred crops, plants in combination can be used such as
   a. tomato plants and basil.
   b. oregano and basil plants.
   c. basil and cabbage plants.
   d. cabbage and tomato plants.

b 　 5/V3

7. Some people have been known to react to the food additive known as MSG by exhibiting symptoms, such as
   a. stomach ulcers.
   b. intense headaches and depression.
   c. muscle pain, especially in the calves.
   d. all of the above.

d | 5/V3 | 8. In order to avoid the adverse side-effects of MSG or other food additives, people should
  a. learn to read labels to find the offensive additive.
  b. eat more fresh fruit, vegetables, and whole grains.
  c. ask that the offensive food additive be left out of foods when eating out.
  d. all of the above.

b | 2/V4 | 9. Time and temperature are two components of safe food handling. The third basic component is
  a. speed.
  b. cleanliness.
  c. frequency.
  d. intensity.

b | 2/V4 | 10. When bacteria on meat is transferred to vegetables that were cut on the same board as the meat, the process is referred to as
  a. sanitation-inhibition.
  b. cross-contamination.
  c. error-in-preparation.
  d. food-irresponsibility.

a | 2/V4 | 11. When handling fruits, vegetables, and meats in the kitchen, the best advice is to
  a. avoid cross-contamination by sanitizing utensils.
  b. keep foods refrigerated until ready to eat, then serve immediately.
  c. avoid taking a bite of raw food unless it's stamped "Safe For Consumption."
  d. wash hands and face immediately after handling meats.

Objective

7/V1 | 12. Sales of soft drinks, beer, and wine have taken a back seat compared to sales of

7/V1 | 13. How can a consumer determine what the source of a bottled water is?

4/V2 | 14. Bat guana is an alternative in organic farming for the use of

| 15. Name one alternative to pesticide use in organic farming.

2/V4 | 16. Transfer of bacteria from one food to another during preparation and handling is known as

2/V4 | 17. One basic component of safe food handling Is

2/V4 | 18. According to the components of safe food handling, the temperature range at which cold food is safest is

Answer

12. bottled water.

13. Read the label.

14. pesticides.

15. Answer may be any of the following:
    * Earthworm castings
    * Bat guana
    * Seedless cow manure
    * Lady bugs
    * Compatible plants

16. cross-contamination.

17. Answer may be any one of the following:
    * time.
    * temperature.
    * sanitation (cleanliness).

18. less than 40 degrees F.

Lesson 26: Applied Nutrition

Ans	Objective		
c	1/V1	1.	The reasons the Pathways subjects chose to participate in the Nutrition Pathways program included all of the following EXCEPT a. a family history of heart disease. b. a family history of diabetes. c. having colon cancer. d. being overweight.
d	1/V1	2.	Of the three subjects who participated in the Nutrition Pathways program, the subject(s) who had the most life threatening condition included the one(s) a. with type II diabetes. b. who was overweight. c. with high blood cholesterol. d. a and c.
d	1/V1	3.	The Pathways subject who had high blood cholesterol was motivated to participate because his father a. had a heart attack when he was 48 years old. b. passed away shortly before the beginning of the program. c. also had high blood cholesterol. d. all of the above.
b	1/V1	4.	The goal of the weight loss subject to lose 40 pounds in one year was completely a. realistic. b. unrealistic. c. achieved. d. b and c.
a	2/V2	5.	Among the reasons why people fail to change nutrition and lifestyle habits include a. setting goals too high. b. changing old habits too slowly. c. having "gotten off the path" then returned. d. all of the above.
d	2/V2	6.	One of the lessons the subject with type II diabetes learned from the program about food intake was that a. deprivation is one reason why people fail at weight loss. b. people can have desserts, but in moderation. c. people must change their attitudes regarding sweets as being off limits. d. all of the above.
c	3/V3	7.	Other factors that can "get in the way" of achieving goals regarding lifestyle and nutrition changes include a. sessions with a health professional. b. taking a course in nutrition. c. jobs and everyday stresses. d. all of the above.

c   3/V3   8. Of the challenges faced by the subject who wanted to lose weight, the most critical to her success was
                              a. managing a child by herself.
                              b. remodeling her home.
                              c. exercising regularly.
                              d. controlling two work-related projects.

c   3/V3   9. The greatest success for the subject who has type II diabetes was
                              a. losing 50 pounds by the end of the year.
                              b. jogging two miles in 20 minutes.
                              c. going from two insulin injections per day to none.
                              d. all of the above.

b   3/V3   10. One of the outcomes of the program for the subject with high blood cholesterol was that he
                              a. was able to stay off of cholesterol-lowering medication.
                              b. had to go back on cholesterol-lowering medication.
                              c. showed significant reductions in HDL and increases in LDL.
                              d. a and c.

d   4/V4   11. The philosophical thread that runs through Nutrition Pathways includes the statement(s)
                              a. "food should be for pleasure as well as nourishment."
                              b. "nutrition and lifestyle is a matter of the right balance."
                              c. "exercise is a critical component of a healthy lifestyle."
                              d. all of the above.

b   4/V4   12. The philosophical emphasis throughout Nutrition Pathways can be best summed up in which one of the following statements?
                              a. "Change your life."
                              b. "Balance your choices."
                              c. "Deprivation breeds success."
                              d. "Variety equals challenge."

Objective

5/V5   13. Describe the importance of exercise with respect to stress reduction and balance in people's lives and its impact on type II diabetes, high blood cholesterol, and overweight.

6/V6   14. What advice would you give to someone who wanted or needed to change nutrition or lifestyle habits? Include comments on the following: the need for evaluation of current physical and/or nutrition status; steps necessary to improve nutrient status or physical status; ways to handle challenges that might interfere with healthful choices; and the importance of balance and moderation in choices.

Answer

13. Answers should include the following points:

*   Exercise is critical for stress reduction as well as the overall success of a sound nutrition program.
*   Exercise provides more energy to tackle the day.
*   Exercise doesn't have to be structured, but must be balanced with good nutrition for success.
*   Type II diabetes will improve with regular exercise because it helps muscles utilize more blood glucose.
*   Exercise may help people with type II diabetes reduce insulin injections or stop them all together.
*   Exercise will help with weight loss better than dieting alone and will help maintain weight once it is lost.
*   Exercise helps HDL cholesterol increase and can reduce LDL cholesterol if done regularly and aerobically.

14. Answers will be highly individualized but should include some of the following points:

*   If the person has a life-threatening condition or disease, they must be evaluated by health care professionals before making changes.
*   Progress slowly for permanent, safe changes.
*   Make changes broad lifestyle changes, not temporary ones that you will discard after achieving your goal.
*   Do not expect perfection from yourself when making changes-- backsliding is to be expected, but get back on track when you discover the slip.
*   Do not deprive yourself of favorite foods--build them into your eating plan and use moderation.
*   Exercise should become a regular, weekly part of your nutrition program for life--not just until you have reached a goal.
*   Keep a positive outlook and attitude--it took years to get this way--it'll take a long time for permanent change.